PLANT-BASED

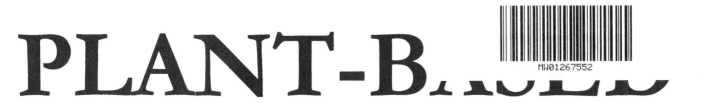

COOKBOOK FOR BEGINNERS

1000 Days of Healthy, Easy, and Quick Recipes to Enjoy Your
New Healthy Lifestyle With Taste

By

KEELY FRANZ

Table Of Contents

Introduction

Have you ever seen or heard of anyone who has lost weight and is looking healthy? Losing weight doesn't always have to be complicated, challenging, and expensive. Eating healthy by following the right diet might not seem like an easy task. But this cookbook will show you how eating plants can be fun and yummy too!

Here are 6 tips:
1. Do not give up on your favorite meat or dairy. You can still eat them occasionally but in smaller portions, as they are high in calories, sodium, and fat content.
2. Eat smaller meals a few times a day. Eat more servings of vegetables, beans, and whole grains that are high in calcium, potassium, iron, and protein.
3. Get rid of all processed foods from your home. Many packaged meals contain processed vegetables and cereals with artificial ingredients.
4. Drink alkaline water throughout the day to help balance your body's pH balance. Do not be too strict on this guideline as it can make you feel drowsy, lethargic, and dehydrated if you do not drink enough water every day.
5. Get lots of relaxation and sleep to aid your body's healing and regeneration. More of the nutrients from your meals will be put to use by your body if you get enough sleep at night.
6. Try out the recipes in this book, and you will notice how delicious it is! As you eat healthier, you will start feeling better and better! Most importantly, being healthy isn't about looking good but also feeling good and having a great life ahead of you.

This article outlines how to start a plant-based diet. The ingredients used in these recipes are completely plant-based, the cooking directions are easy to follow, and the preparation time is short.
Have fun cooking and have a healthier life!

Chapter 1: What Is A Plant-Based Diet?

Macrobiotic Plant-Based Diet

George, a Japanese philosopher, was the first to invent the term macrobiotic. However, macrobiotics did not become popular in the United States until the 1960s. Macrobiotics is a lifestyle that emphasizes balance and stability. Macrobiotics is based on the habits and practices of long-established global civilizations that have avoided chronic sickness for millennia. Its goal is to achieve a healthy balance of physical and mental well-being. Whole grains, legumes, vegetables, nuts, seeds, fruits, and naturally pickled & fermented foods are all part of the macrobiotic plant-based diet. In addition, meat, dairy, artificial components, and processed foods are eliminated or reduced.

Macrobiotic Diet Benefits

A macrobiotic diet has several health advantages. Fiber, nutrients, and minerals are abundant in plant-based diets. As a result, a nutritious plant-based diet helps in bodily balance, improved stomach and digestion, immunity, and toxin elimination.

High blood pressure, diabetes, & hypoglycemia may all be prevented by eating a diet rich in vegetables and whole grains. These meals are well-balanced and consistent. As a result, they aid in the maintenance of your blood pressure. In addition, plant-based meals help with weight control and enhance body functioning; therefore, the macrobiotic diet lowers the risk of cardiovascular disease.

If you eat a processed-food-heavy diet, your heart does not have to work as hard. Fatigue - Today's diet is excessively acidic and unbalanced. As a result, providing oxygen to vital organs becomes more challenging for the body. Furthermore, the digestive tract has difficulty absorbing nutrients and minerals. As a result, your body begins to recover and regenerate when you transition to a plant-based diet. You will feel more invigorated, younger, and stronger as a result of this treatment.

Vegan Lifestyle

Vegans take charge with purpose. No matter how modest, they make every effort to build a world where no animals are hurt by human service. And it's not just about food. Vegans have been at the forefront of several demonstrations against circus performances and other forms of entertainment that compel animals to act for human pleasure. A circus has nothing to do with Nutrition Facts per Servings (unless popcorn and cotton candy are included) but all to do with animal welfare. Animals compelled to act for human pleasure often exhibit no evidence of enjoyment or desire to do so. As a result, trainers must use pain to elicit the correct behavior from the animal.

Veganism entails consciously avoiding any behavior that harms animal welfare.

Veganism

It is an ideology and way of life that opposes the use of other creatures for personal gain. We're all here for a reason, and non-human species contribute just as much to our environment as humans do. Vegans think that rather than living as "apex predators," mankind can coexist with animals. Instead of imposing our will on animals, we may help them live as naturally as possible. The vegan diet is an integral aspect of the lifestyle. Vegans will not eat eggs, dairy, meat, or any other animal byproduct, even bee honey. But it's a lot more than that. Animals are employed in producing a wide range of consumer goods cosmetics, including soaps and apparel. Vegans, for example, use synthetic textiles rather than wool from llamas, alpacas, sheep, and other animals. These animals aren't killed for their fur, to be sure. They are, however, afraid of the shearing process, which they do not understand, and are deprived of their natural protection from the elements. Veganism is all about intention, but it's also about being conscious. Before purchasing anything from the store, a vegan considers whether it has a detrimental impact on animals.

Pros and Cons of Plant-Based Diet

PROS

- Protection from certain types of cancer

- Improved glycemic control (reduction of Hemoglobin A1C in people with Diabetes Type II)
- Weight management
- Lower total cholesterol and LDL levels
- Improved neurocognitive performance, dementia prevention, and Alzheimer's disease management
- Reduced carbon footprint
- Lower risk of developing diabetes type II
- Cardiovascular health has improved (decreased blood pressure, lowered heart rate, reduced risk for cardiovascular events)

CONS

There are several methods to consume a plant-based diet that are harmful. In addition to boosting plant products, the research on the advantages of a plant-based diet stresses fresh, complete components and reducing processed meals. Changing to a plant-based diet or just adding more fresh food to one's diet can undoubtedly enhance one's health. Plant-based diets, on the other hand, may entail the following health risks if they are not properly planned and educated about foods:

- Low calcium and vitamin D consumption leads to decreased bone mineralization and an increased risk of fractures.
- Lower essential fatty acid intake
- Iron deficiency
- Low protein intake
- Vitamin B12 deficiency

Difference Between Vegan and Vegetarian Diet

What Is a Vegan Diet?

A vegan diet forbids the use of both animal protein and animal products. Meat, shellfish, dairy, milk, eggs, cheese, and honey are all examples. A vegan diet may also be tailored to the individual.
For example, someone may abstain from using animal-tested cosmetics due to animal welfare and rights concerns. Instead, choose a raw vegan diet and eat largely uncooked and unprocessed foods for health reasons.

What Is a Vegetarian Diet?

A vegetarian diet avoids animal protein and meat, comparable to a vegan diet.
The difference between a vegan and a vegetarian diet is that a vegetarian diet may include animal products such as milk, dairy, cheese, eggs, and honey.

What Is a Macrobiotic Diet and Lifestyle?

A macrobiotic definition is a concept of holistic principles & dynamic practices that direct nutritional, physical, mental, social, & environmental health through choices in diet, exercise, and lifestyle. As a result, you may be a macrobiotic vegan or vegetarian, but being vegetarian or vegan does not imply a macrobiotic.

Benefits

Why Plant-Based?

Maintaining a healthy weight is easier with a plant-based diet. One of the essential things you can do to lower your cancer risk is to maintain a healthy weight. The only thing more essential than keeping a healthy weight for cancer prevention is not smoking.
It is because being overweight induces inflammation as well as hormone imbalances. If you're overweight or obese, you're more likely to get colorectal, postmenopausal breast, uterine, esophageal, kidney, and pancreatic cancers, to name a few.
Many things that cause weight gain are eliminated when you largely eat vegetables. When you add exercise to the mix, you're on your way to losing weight.
Fiber is abundant in plants. All raw plant foods include fiber. It's what gives the plant its structure, and eating more of it gives you access to a slew of advantages.
Eating a plant-based diet enhances gut health, allowing you to absorb more nutrients from the food that help your immune system and decrease inflammation.

Fiber may help decrease cholesterol and blood sugar levels, and it's also beneficial for intestinal health.

Fiber is crucial in lowering your cancer risk. It is particularly true if you're at risk for colorectal cancer, the third most prevalent cancer. A plant-based diet also decreases your chances of contracting other ailments. However, the advantages of eating primarily vegetables go beyond lowering your cancer risk.

A plant-based diet has also been demonstrated to lower the risk of heart disease, stroke, diabetes, and some mental diseases.

List of the Most Common Vegetarian Practices

Fruitarian

A fruitarian is someone who lives on a diet composed primarily or exclusively of fruits, nuts, and seeds. They might eat vegetables but not in as significant quantities as other types of vegetarians, depending on the intensity of their fruitarian lifestyle. Many fruitarians follow a completely vegan diet, eating no animal byproducts, including meat and dairy products. However, there is no standardization in these terms. Like vegans, the fruitarian will not consume any form of meat or dairy, but the vast majority of these people consume eggs and honey. More moderate and less strict fruitarians may eat small amounts of eggs and/or honey.

Vegan

What does it mean to be vegan? A vegan is someone who chooses not to consume (or use) any animal products whatsoever; this includes any meat (including poultry), dairy products, eggs, or honey—even if they are organic or local. Vegans generally avoid products that have been tested on animals, even products that are labeled as vegetarian. There is so much to learn about the vegan lifestyle. Not only is it a diet that does not harm animals, but it's also one that excludes all animal products—meat, dairy, and eggs. There are many types of veganism with varying degrees of strictness, but they're all relatively similar in their environmental impact and ethical values.

Lacto-Vegetarian

A Lacto-vegetarian is someone who's not a vegetarian but still eats dairy and eggs. They sometimes also eat meat that comes from animals that were raised on farms by humans. What does being dairy and egg-free have to do with cooking? Since they aren't vegetarians, Lacto-vegetarians are more than willing to experiment with different types of meat or animal products. This makes them excellent for persons who wish to experiment with veganism as well as those who like the flexibility to eat delicacies like bacon without feeling bad.

Being a Lacto-vegetarian can also make it much easier to be vegan. Many lacto-vegetarians and vegans have found they can use eggs, cheese, and dairy substitutes to replicate many foods that would typically contain meat. That way, they can enjoy some of the same foods while not really needing to deal with tasting or eating meat.

Lacto-Ovo-Vegetarian

You'll be incorporating plenty of fruits, veggies, whole grains, nuts, and seeds, but cheese and eggs are also included in this well-balanced food plan.

That means it's perfect for people who are used to eating animal protein but don't want to give up their favorite foods. It's also a great diet if you're an advocate for healthy eating but need to cut down on animal protein consumption.

Peach-Vegetarian

A strict vegan will exclude all animal by-products such as eggs, dairy, and honey. A vegetarian will exclude red meat and poultry but not fish or eggs. A peach-vegetarian would eliminate red meat, poultry, dairy, and fish from their diet but still, consume eggs and honey.

The term 'peach' reflects the idea that people who have chosen this type of diet might pursue a more pleasurable vegetarian lifestyle because they are open to eating foods that many vegetarians find off-limits—namely fruits such as peaches. The word 'vegetarian' refers to this lifestyle, not the food that a person eats.

Partially-Vegetarian

A partially vegetarian diet hinges on the level of consumption of animal flesh. Some people adopt this type of diet to reduce their intake of animal protein while maintaining a non-vegan lifestyle for other reasons or as a transitional step to veganism. People who follow a partially-vegetarian diet include pescatarians, lacto-ovo-vegetarians, and lacto-vegetarians. Each of these categories is based on the level of animal consumption that the individual engages in. The decision to adopt a partially-vegetarian diet is usually made for health reasons such as lower cholesterol levels or weight loss.

In fact, over two-thirds of adults in the United States are either vegetarians or have reduced their meat consumption. Nowadays, vegetarianism is not just for weight loss; it has become a way to change your life and make a powerful statement about sustainability. However, the majority of people are unsure how to maintain this lifestyle without creating substantial dietary deprivation.

The Vegetarian Resource Group states that anyone who is vegetarian and works out daily should consume a minimum of 2000 calories a day. With that said, if you're eating meatless meals five days a week, that leaves you with 2200 calories to add to your diet every day. If you are following the [Fruitarian Diet], which is essentially all fruit, 100% of those calories should come from fruits/vegetables. In addition, according to the Fruitarian Diet website, a fruitarian's caloric needs can be met by eating about 150-250 grams of fruit each day.

While this diet plan is one of the more restrictive ones featured on this site, it can be done with little to no exercise. However, depending on your current weight and exercise program, you may need to limit the number of calories you consume only from fruit.

If you're already on a strict vegan or vegetarian diet and want to try becoming fully fruitarian, you should slowly transition into the diet over several weeks. However, if you don't feel comfortable eating a completely raw diet (most people don't), cooked foods such as stews and smoothies are allowed on this diet as long as they are derived primarily from fruit.

Daily Exercise: 15 Minutes for Day

1. Walk-Out Push-Up

This technique, according to Watkins, engages numerous muscle groups and includes different planes of movement, increasing heart rate. Begin by standing with the feet about hip-width apart. Bend forward at the hips and bring the hands to the floor slowly. Slowly move your hands forward after they've touched the floor until the spine is straight and you're in the push-up beginning position. Complete a complete push-up, then walk the hands back to the feet and carefully roll the spine up 1 vertebra at a time to return to standing.

2. Standard Squat

Squats compel the brain to participate actively. To concentrate on equal weight distribution between the left and right leg; to maintain the chest-high & back straight; to activate the glutes; to halt at the change of direction to prevent momentum from accumulating, and to stand with full extension of the hips.

3. Jumping Jacks

The age-old jumping jack causes a lot of folks to roll their eyes. However, a sprinkle of plyometrics is quite advantageous when it comes to functional fitness. As a consequence of living in shoes and being sedentary, neurotransmitters in the feet become drowsy. The light impact is a terrific way to get those wacky animals to wake up. When done correctly, the jacks, like the walk-outs, activate various muscular groups and raise the heart rate.

4. Hip Bridge

A degree of happiness for everybody. Furthermore, like with the squat, your brain is actively involved in this movement. Foot positioning, weight distribution, and breathing are crucial. Another aspect of this regulated proprioception is maintaining the toes on the floor. When your heels take all of the body weight, the lower back is put under extra strain. On the other hand, the hamstrings and glutes engage and help extend the hips when the body shifts direction while the toes remain down.

Chapter 2: Breakfast & Smoothies

Coconut Blackberry Breakfast Bowl

Preparation Time: 15 minutes
Cooking Time: 2 minutes
Servings: 2
Ingredients:

- 2 tablespoons chia seeds
- ¼ cup coconut flakes
- 1 cup spinach
- ¼ cup water
- 3 tablespoons ground flaxseed
- 1 cup unsweetened coconut milk
- 1 cup blackberries

Apple Avocado Coconut Smoothie

Preparation Time: 5 minutes
Cooking Time: 0 minutes
Servings: 2
Ingredients:

- 1 teaspoon coconut oil
- 1 tablespoon collagen powder
- 1 tablespoon fresh lime juice
- ½ cup unsweetened coconut milk
- ¼ apple, slice
- 1 avocado

Directions:

1. Add all elements into the blender and mix until smooth and creamy.
2. Serve and enjoy.

Nutrition:

- Calories: 262
- Fat: 23.9 g
- Carbohydrates: 13.6 g
- Protein: 2 g

Chia Cinnamon Smoothie

Preparation Time: 5 minutes
Cooking Time: 0 minutes
Servings: 1
Ingredients:

- 2 scoops vanilla protein powder
- 1 tablespoon chia seeds
- ½ teaspoon cinnamon
- 1 tablespoon coconut oil
- ½ cup water
- ½ cup unsweetened coconut milk

Directions:

Directions:

1. Add blackberries, flaxseed, spinach, and coconut milk into the blender and mix until smooth. Fry coconut flakes in the pan for 1–2 minutes.
2. Pour berry mixture into the serving bowls, then sprinkle coconut flakes and chia seeds on top.
3. Serve immediately and enjoy.

Nutrition:

- Calories: 182
- Fat: 11.4 g
- Carbohydrates: 14.5 g
- Protein: 5.3 g

1. Add all elements into the blender and mix until smooth and creamy.
2. Serve immediately and enjoy.

Nutrition:

- Calories: 397
- Fat: 23.9 g
- Carbohydrates: 13.4 g
- Protein: 31.6 g

Avocado Choco Cinnamon Smoothie

Preparation Time: 5 minutes
Cooking Time: 0 minutes
Servings: 1
Ingredients:

- ½ teaspoon coconut oil
- 5 drops liquid stevia
- ¼ teaspoon vanilla extract
- 1 teaspoon ground cinnamon
- 2 teaspoons unsweetened cocoa powder
- ½ avocado
- ¾ cup unsweetened coconut milk

Directions:

1. Add all elements into the blender and mix until smooth and creamy.
2. Serve immediately and enjoy.

Nutrition:

- Calories: 95 Fat: 8.3 g
- Carbohydrates: 5.1 g Protein: 1.2 g

Acai Bowl

Preparation Time: 5 minutes
Cooking Time: 0 minutes
Servings: 1
Ingredients:

- 1 packet frozen Sambazon acai berries

- ½ cup strawberries
- 1 ripe banana
- 1 teaspoon maple syrup
- ½ cup almond milk

Optional toppings:
- Fruit slices
- Dried fruit
- Shredded coconut
- Granola

Directions:
1. Mix all ingredients in a high-speed blender until smooth.
2. Pour in a bowl and top with fresh or dried fruit, nuts, seeds, or granola.

Nutrition:
- Calories: 296
- Fat: 3 g
- Carbohydrates: 66 g
- Protein: 7 g

Peanut Butter Oat Bars

Preparation Time: 15 minutes
Cooking Time: 30 minutes
Servings: 8
Ingredients:
- ¼ cup almond milk
- 2 tablespoons maple syrup
- ½ cup peanut butter
- ¼ teaspoon sea salt
- 2 cups old-fashioned rolled oats

Directions:
1. Preheat oven to 350°Fahrenheit. Prepare a 9x9 baking dish lined using parchment paper. Mix all the ingredients, except for the rolled oats, together in a large bowl.
2. Add in the rolled oats and mix them. Place and spread the oat mixture into the baking dish and bake for 30 minutes. Cool for about 10 to 20 minutes. Cut into 8 serving bars.

Nutrition:
- Calories: 189
- Fat: 10 g
- Carbohydrates: 21 g
- Protein: 7 g

Pumpkin Spice Oat Bars

Preparation Time: 15 minutes
Cooking Time: 40 minutes
Servings: 8
Ingredients:
- 1 cup pumpkin puree
- ½ cup unsweetened applesauce

- ½ cup maple syrup
- 1 teaspoon vanilla extract
- 2 cups old-fashioned rolled oats
- 2 teaspoons pumpkin pie spice
- ¼ teaspoon sea salt
- ½ cup dried cranberries
- ¼ cup pistachio nuts, chopped

Directions:
1. Preheat oven to 350°Fahrenheit. Prepare a 9x9 baking dish lined using parchment paper. Whisk together pumpkin puree, applesauce, maple syrup, and vanilla until smooth.
2. Stir in the rolled oats, pumpkin pie spice, and salt. Once oats are moistened, add in the cranberries and pistachio nuts.
3. Place and spread the oat mixture into the baking dish and bake for 40 minutes or until golden brown. Cool for about 10 to 20 minutes. Cut into 8 serving bars.

Nutrition:
- Calories: 186
- Fat: 3 g
- Carbohydrates: 37 g
- Protein: 4 g

Sweet Breakfast Rice

Preparation Time: 10 minutes
Cooking Time: 5 minutes
Servings: 4
Ingredients:
- 1-½ cups almond milk
- 1-½ cups cooked brown rice
- ½ cup raisins
- 3 ounces shredded coconut
- 1 pear, diced
- 1 apple, diced
- 1 tablespoon maple syrup
- 1 teaspoon cinnamon

Directions:
1. Mix all elements in a saucepan and heat through.
2. Serve immediately.

Nutrition:
- Calories: 267
- Fat: 4 g
- Carbohydrates: 54 g
- Protein: 6 g

Banana Walnut Chia Cereal

Preparation Time: 15 minutes
Cooking Time: 0 minutes
Servings: 1

Ingredients:

- 6 ounces almond milk
- 2 tablespoons chia seeds
- 1 ripe banana, chopped
- 1 tablespoon walnuts, chopped
- ½ teaspoon cinnamon
- 1 tablespoon maple syrup

Directions:

1. Soak your chia seeds in almond milk for approximately 5 minutes.
2. Add in bananas, walnuts, and cinnamon.
3. Drizzle with maple syrup.
4. Serve.

Nutrition:

- Calories: 376
- Fat: 13 g
- Carbohydrates: 60 g
- Protein: 10 g

Broccoli Quiche

Preparation Time: 10 minutes
Cooking Time: 10 minutes
Servings: 1
Ingredients:

- 1 egg
- 1 tablespoon cheddar cheese, grated
- 4 broccoli florets
- 3 tablespoons heavy cream
- Salt and pepper to taste

Directions:

1. Grease 5-inch quiche dish with cooking spray.
2. In a bowl, whisk the egg with cheese, cream, pepper, and salt. Add broccoli and stir well.
3. Pour egg mixture into the quiche dish.
4. Place dish into the Air Fryer basket and cook at 325°Fahrenheit for 10 minutes.
5. Serve

Nutrition:

- Calories: 173
- Fat: 13 g
- Carbohydrates: 6.5 g
- Sugar 1.9 g
- Protein: 9.9 g
- Cholesterol 191 mg

Broccoli Fritters

Preparation Time: 10 minutes
Cooking Time: 15 minutes
Servings: 4
Ingredients:

- 3 cups broccoli florets, steam and chopped

- 2 cups cheddar cheese, shredded
- ¼ cup almond flour
- 2 eggs, lightly beaten
- 2 garlic cloves, minced

Directions:

1. Line Air Fryer basket with parchment paper.
2. Add all ingredients into the mixing bowl and blend until well combined.
3. Make patties from the broccoli mixture and place them in the Air Fryer basket.
4. Cook at 375°Fahrenheit for 15 minutes. Turn patties halfway through.
5. Serve

Nutrition:

- Calories: 285
- Fat: 22 g
- Carbohydrates: 6.3 g
- Sugar 1.7 g
- Protein: 19.2 g
- Cholesterol 141 mg

Spicy Brussels Sprouts

Preparation Time: 10 minutes
Cooking Time: 14 minutes
Servings: 2
Ingredients:

- ½ pound Brussels sprouts, trimmed and halved
- 1 tablespoon chives, chopped
- ¼ teaspoon cayenne
- ½ teaspoon chili powder
- ½ tablespoon olive oil

Directions:

1. Add all ingredients into the large bowl and toss well.
2. Spread Brussels sprouts in the Air Fryer basket and cook at 370°Fahrenheit for 14 minutes. Shake basket halfway through.
3. Serve

Nutrition:

- Calories: 82
- Fat: 4.1 g
- Carbohydrates: 10.9 g
- Sugar 2.6 g
- Protein: 4 g
- Cholesterol 0 mg

Zucchini Breakfast Patties

Preparation Time: 10 minutes
Cooking Time: 15 minutes
Servings: 6
Ingredients:

- 1 cup zucchini, shredded, and squeeze out all liquid
- 2 tablespoons onion, minced
- 1 egg, lightly beaten
- ¼ teaspoon red pepper flakes
- ¼ cup parmesan cheese, grated

Directions:
1. Add all ingredients into the bowl and mix until well combined.
2. Make small patties from the zucchini mixture and place them into the Air Fryer basket.
3. Cook at 400°Fahrenheit for 15 minutes.
4. Serve

Nutrition:
- Calories: 48
- Fat: 3.3 g
- Carbohydrates: 2.1 g
- Sugar 0.7 g
- Protein: 3.1 g
- Cholesterol 31 mg

Spinach & Ricotta Cups

Preparation Time: 10 minutes
Cooking Time: 10 minutes
Servings: 2
Ingredients:
- 2 large eggs
- 2 tablespoons heavy cream
- 2 tablespoons frozen spinach, thawed
- 4 teaspoons ricotta cheese, crumbled
- Salt and freshly ground black pepper, to taste

Directions:
1. Grease 2 ramekins.
2. In each ramekin, crack one egg.
3. Divide the cream spinach, cheese, salt, and black pepper in each ramekin and gently stir to mix without breaking the yolks.
4. Turn the "Temperature Knob" of Power XL Air Fryer Grill to line the temperature to 330°Fahrenheit.
5. Turn the "Function Knob" to settle on "Air Fry."
6. Turn the "Timer Knob" to line the time for 10 minutes.
7. After preheating, arrange the ramekins pan over the roasting rack.
8. Insert the roasting rack at position 2 of the Air Fryer Grill.
9. When the cooking time is over, remove the ramekins and place them onto a wire rack to chill for five minutes before serving.

Nutrition:
- Calories: 138

- Fat: 11.4 g
- Carbohydrates: 1.4 g
- Protein: 7.8 g

Breakfast Radish Hash Browns

Preparation Time: 10 minutes
Cooking Time: 13 minutes
Servings: 2
Ingredients:
- 1 pound radishes, clean and sliced
- 1 onion, sliced
- 1 tablespoon olive oil
- 1 teaspoon onion powder
- 1 teaspoon garlic powder
- ½ teaspoon paprika
- ¼ teaspoon pepper
- ½ teaspoon salt

Directions:
1. Toss sliced radishes and onion with olive oil.
2. Grease Air Fryer basket with cooking spray.
3. Put radish and onion mixture into the Air Fryer basket and cook at 360°Fahrenheit for 8 minutes.
4. Transfer radish and onion mixture into the mixing bowl. Add onion powder, garlic powder, paprika, pepper, and salt; then toss well.
5. Return radish and onion mixture into the Air Fryer basket and cook for 5 minutes more.
6. Serve and enjoy.

Nutrition:
- Calories: 125
- Fat: 7.4 g
- Carbohydrates: 13.6 g
- Sugar 3.2 g
- Protein: 3.6 g
- Cholesterol 0 mg

Breakfast Strata

Preparation Time: 6 hours
Cooking Time: 2 hours
Servings: 8
Ingredients:
- 18 eggs
- 2 packs croutons
- 1 pack cheddar
- Salt and pepper, to taste
- 1 pack chopped spinach
- 3 cups milk
- 3 cups chopped ham
- 1 jar red peppers

Directions:

1. Preheat the Power XL Air Fryer Grill to 135°Celsius or 275°Fahrenheit.
2. Grease the pan with a non-stick spray.
3. Spread layers of ham, spinach, cheese, and croutons, and red peppers.
4. Pour eggs mixed with milk and seasoning in the pan and refrigerate.
5. Bake for 2 hours and leave to rest for 15 minutes.

Nutrition:
- Calories: 140
- Carbohydrates: 6 g
- Protein: 16 g
- Fat: 5 g

Sheet Pan Shakshuka

Preparation Time: 15 minutes
Cooking Time: 10 minutes
Servings: 4
Ingredients:
- 4 large eggs
- 1 large Anaheim chili, chopped
- 2 tablespoons vegetable oil
- ½ cup onion, chopped
- 1 teaspoon cumin, ground
- 2 minced garlic cloves
- ½ cup feta cheese
- ½ teaspoon paprika
- 1 can tomatoes
- Salt and pepper to taste

Directions:
1. Saute the chili and onions in vegetable oil until tender.
2. Pour in the remaining ingredients except for eggs and cook until thick.
3. Make 4 pockets to pour in the eggs.
4. Bake for 10 minutes at 191°Celsius or 375°Fahrenheit in the Power XL Air Fryer Grill.
5. Top it off with feta.

Nutrition:
- Calories: 219
- Carbohydrates: 20 g
- Protein: 10 g
- Fat: 11 g

Coconut-Blueberry Cereal

Preparation Time: 20 minutes
Cooking Time: 20 minutes
Servings: 4
Ingredients:
- ½ cup dried blueberries

- ½ cup unsweetened coconut flakes
- 1 cup pumpkin seeds
- 2 cups chopped pecans
- 6 medium dates, pitted
- ⅓ cup coconut oil
- 2 teaspoons cinnamon
- ½ teaspoon sea salt

Directions:
1. Add coconut oil, dates, and half the pecans to a food processor; pulse until finely ground.
2. Add pumpkin seeds and the remaining pecans, then continue pulsing until roughly chopped.
3. Transfer the mixture to a large bowl and add cinnamon, vanilla and salt; spread on a baking sheet/pan that can fit in your foodie air fry toaster oven and set on bake at 320°Fahrenheit for about 22 minutes or until browned.
4. Remove from the foodie air fry toaster oven and let cool slightly before stirring in blueberries and coconut.
5. Enjoy!

Nutrition:
- Calories: 372 Carbohydrates: 12 g
- Fat: 25.2 g Protein: 20.1 g

Air Toasted French Toast

Preparation Time: 5 minutes
Cooking Time: 20 minutes
Servings: 3
Ingredients:
- 6 slices preferred bread
- ¾ cup milk
- 3 eggs
- 1 teaspoon pure vanilla extract
- 1 tablespoon ground cinnamon
- Maple syrup for serving

Directions:
1. Combine all the ingredients apart from the bread in a medium bowl until well mixed.
2. Dunk each slice of bread into the egg mix. Gently shake the excess off and place in a greased pan.
3. Air toast in the fryer for 6 minutes.
4. To serve, drizzle with maple syrup.

Nutrition:
- Calories: 245
- Carbohydrates: 28.5 g
- Fat: 7.5 g
- Protein: 14.9 g

French Toast

Preparation Time: 5 minutes

Cooking Time: 10 minutes
Servings: 4
Ingredients:

- 2 slices bread
- 1 teaspoon liquid vanilla
- 3 eggs
- 1 tablespoon Margarine

Directions:

1. Preheat the Power XL Air Fryer Grill by setting it to toast/pizza mode.
2. Adjust the temperature to 375°Fahrenheit; insert the pizza tray.
3. In a bowl, whisk the eggs and vanilla.
4. Spread the margarine on the bread. Transfer it into the egg and allow to soak.
5. Place on the Power XL Air Fryer pizza rack and set time to 6 minutes. Flip after 3 minutes.
6. Serve and enjoy.

Serving Suggestions: Serve topped with yogurt and honey.
Nutrition:

- Calories: 99
- Fat: 0.2 g
- Carbohydrates: 7 g
- Proteins 5 g

Raspberry Oatmeal

Preparation Time: 10 minutes
Cooking Time: 20 minutes
Servings: 4
Ingredients:

- 1 cup shredded coconut
- 2 teaspoons stevia
- 1 teaspoon cinnamon powder
- 2 cups almond milk
- ½ cup raspberries

Directions:

1. Mix all the ingredients in a bowl.
2. Pour into the Air Fryer baking pan.
3. Transfer to the Power XL Air Fryer Grill.
4. Using the knob, select bake/pizza mode.
5. Adjust the temperature to 360°Fahrenheit.
6. Bake for 15 minutes.
7. Serve and enjoy.

Serving Suggestions: Garnish with coconut.
Nutrition:

- Calories: 172
- Fat: 5 g
- Carbohydrates: 5 g
- Proteins 6 g

Zucchini Fritters

Preparation Time: 8 minutes

Cooking Time: 20 minutes
Servings: 4
Ingredients:

- 10 ounces zucchini
- 7 ounces halloumi cheese
- 2 eggs
- ¼ cup all-purpose flour
- 1 teaspoon dried dill
- Salt and black pepper to taste

Directions:

1. Preheat the Power XL Air Fryer Grill by selecting bake/pizza mode.
2. Adjust temperature to 360°Fahrenheit and time to 5 minutes.
3. In a bowl, mix all the ingredients.
4. Make small fritters from the mixture.
5. Place them on the Air fryer baking tray.
6. Transfer into the Power XL Air Fryer Grill.
7. Bake for 7 minutes.
8. Serve and enjoy!

Serving Suggestions: Serve with vegetable salad.
Nutrition:

- Calories: 170
- Fat: 15 g
- Carbohydrates: 7 g
- Proteins 12 g

Berry Buckwheat Breakfast Bake

Preparation Time: 15 minutes
Cooking Time: 30 minutes
Servings: 6
Ingredients:

- 1 cup buckwheat flour
- 2 tablespoons flax meal
- ½ teaspoon cinnamon
- ½ teaspoon baking soda
- ¼ teaspoon sea salt
- ½ cup unsweetened almond milk
- ½ cup maple syrup
- 1 teaspoon vanilla extract
- 1 ripe banana
- 1 cup mixed berries

Directions:

1. Preheat oven to 350°Fahrenheit. Prepare a 9x9 baking dish lined using parchment paper. Combine the dry ingredients in a large bowl.
2. In a separate bowl, mix the almond milk, maple syrup, and vanilla extract. Mix the liquid with the dry ingredients.

3. Mash up the banana and stir into the mixture. Blend in the berries. Pour mixture into baking dish. Bake for approximately 30 minutes. Top with fresh fruit or maple syrup.

Nutrition:
- Calories: 221
- Fat: 2 g
- Carbohydrates: 49 g
- Protein: 5 g

Hash Brown Cakes

Preparation Time: 15 minutes
Cooking Time: 10 minutes
Servings: 4
Ingredients:
- 2 potatoes, peeled and grated
- ½ small onion, diced
- ¼ cup whole wheat flour
- 1 tablespoon nutritional yeast
- ½ teaspoon sea salt
- Black pepper to taste

Directions:
1. Peel and coarsely shred potatoes using a grater or in a food processor.
2. Rinse with cold water in your colander, then drain well and then pat dry with paper towels.
3. Place potatoes in a large bowl. Stir in the onions, flour, nutritional yeast, salt, and pepper. Combine well. Preheat a large non-stick skillet over medium heat.
4. For each cake, scoop ¼ of the potato mixture onto the skillet. Press down the potato batter with a spatula to flatten evenly. Cook within 5 minutes.
5. Using a wide spatula, carefully turn potato cakes. Cook again within 3 to 5 minutes more or until golden brown.

Nutrition:
- Calories: 110
- Fat: 0 g
- Carbohydrates: 24 g
- Protein: 4 g

Gorgeous Green Smoothie

Preparation Time: 5 minutes
Cooking Time: 0 minutes
Servings: 2
Ingredients:
- ¼ cup nut or seed butter
- 2 frozen bananas, peeled
- 4 cups tightly packed shredded leafy greens
- 2 tablespoons chia seeds

Directions:
1. Combine all the fixings in a blender and add 3 cups of water. Puree for 30 seconds to 1 minute, until most of the green flecks have disappeared and the texture is smooth and creamy.

Nutrition:
- Calories: 380
- Fat: 22 g
- Protein: 12 g
- Carbohydrates: 41 g

The Berry-Blend Bowl

Preparation Time: 5 minutes
Cooking Time: 0 minutes
Servings: 2
Ingredients:
- 2 cups unsweetened soy milk
- 1 cup frozen blueberries
- 1 cup frozen pitted cherries
- 2 bananas, sliced
- 1 cup maple muesli or granola
- 4 tablespoons hemp seeds

Directions:
1. In a blender, combine the soy milk, blueberries, and cherries. Then puree until smooth. Divide the puree between two serving bowls.
2. Arrange the banana slices halfway around the edge of each bowl. Spoon ½ cup of maple muesli into the center of each bowl.
3. Spoon 2 tablespoons of hemp seeds around the edge of each bowl, opposite the bananas, and serve.

Nutrition:
- Calories: 540
- Fat: 18 g
- Protein: 17 g
- Carbohydrates: 84 g

Fruity Yogurt Parfait

Preparation Time: 5 minutes
Cooking Time: 0 minutes
Servings: 2
Ingredients:
- 2 cups plain plant-based yogurt or cashew cream
- 2 cups fresh blueberries or raspberries
- 1 cup maple muesli or granola
- ¼ teaspoon ground cinnamon

Directions:
1. In an individual serving bowl or parfait glass. Layer ½ cup of yogurt, 1 cup of berries, ½ cup

of muesli, another ½ cup of yogurt, and $^1/_8$ a teaspoon of cinnamon.

2. Repeat in a second serving bowl or parfait glass.

Nutrition:
- Calories: 520
- Fat: 30 g
- Protein: 14 g
- Carbohydrates: 71 g

Apple Avocado Toast

Preparation Time: 5 minutes
Cooking Time: 2 minutes
Servings: 4
Ingredients:
- 1 large ripe avocado, halved and pitted
- 1 small apple, cored
- 2 tablespoons lemon juice
- ½ cup chopped pecans
- ½ teaspoon ground cinnamon
- 4 slices whole-grain bread, toasted

Directions:
1. Scoop your avocado flesh into a small bowl, then mash it with a fork. Cut the apple into $^1/_8$ inch cubes and add them to the avocado.
2. Add the lemon juice, pecans, and cinnamon and gently fold with a rubber spatula until well combined.
3. Spread about ¼ cup of the apple-avocado mixture onto each slice of toast and serve.

Nutrition:
- Calories: 276
- Fat: 19 g
- Protein: 7 g
- Carbohydrates: 25 g

Go-To Grits

Preparation Time: 5 minutes
Cooking Time: 20 minutes
Servings: 4
Ingredients:
- 1 cup cornmeal
- ¼ cup nutritional yeast
- 2 tablespoons lemon juice
- ½ teaspoon salt, or 1 teaspoon spicy umami blend

Directions:
1. In a large saucepan, bring 4 cups of water to a boil over high heat. Lower the heat to medium-high and slowly whisk in the cornmeal. Cook, stirring continuously, until it thickens, about 15 minutes.
2. Stir in the nutritional yeast, lemon juice, and salt. Serve immediately.

Nutrition:
- Calories: 127
- Fat: 1 g
- Protein: 5 g
- Carbohydrates: 25 g

Oatmeal-Raisin Breakfast Bowl

Preparation Time: 5 minutes
Cooking Time: 30 minutes
Servings: 4
Ingredients:
- 1 cup steel-cut oats
- 2 cups unsweetened plant-based milk
- ½ cup raisins
- 1 teaspoon ground cinnamon
- ¼ cup chopped pitted dates
- ¼ cup chopped pecans

Directions:
1. Mix the oats, milk, raisins, and cinnamon in a large saucepan and boil over medium-high heat.
2. Adjust the heat to low, then simmer, occasionally stirring, until the oats are tender, about 25 minutes. Remove from the heat. Stir in the dates and pecans, then serve.

Nutrition:
- Calories: 355
- Fat: 9 g
- Protein: 10 g
- Carbohydrates: 61 g

Cheesy Jackfruit Chilaquiles

Preparation Time: 5 minutes
Cooking Time: 20 minutes
Servings: 4
Ingredients:
- 4 (6-inch) corn tortillas, each cut into 8 strips
- 3 tablespoons aquafaba
- 1 (14-½ ounces) can diced tomatoes
- 1 cup vegetable broth
- 4 garlic cloves
- 1 teaspoon chili powder
- 1 teaspoon cayenne pepper
- 1 teaspoon ground cumin
- 1 teaspoon dried Mexican oregano
- 1 (14 ounces) can jackfruit, drained
- 1 cup cheesy chickpea sauce

Directions:
1. Preheat the oven to 350°Fahrenheit. Prepare your baking sheet lined using parchment paper or a silicone baking mat.
2. In a bowl, combine the tortillas and aquafaba and toss until the strips are completely coated.

Place the tortillas in a single layer on the prepared baking sheet and bake for 15 minutes.

3. In a blender, combine the tomatoes, broth, chili powder, cayenne pepper, cumin, oregano, and puree. Pour the mixture into a large skillet and bring to a boil over medium-high heat.
4. Add the jackfruit to the sauce and return the sauce to a boil. Lower the heat to medium. Add the tortilla strips, gently stir until coated, cover, and cook until the tortillas are slightly soft but still crunchy, 2 to 3 minutes more.

5. Spoon into four bowls. Drizzle about ½ cup of the chickpea sauce over each bowl, if desired, and serve.

Nutrition:

- Calories: 253
- Fat: 3 g
- Protein: 8 g
- Carbohydrates: 52 g

Chapter 3:   Soups & Salads

Cabbage & Beet Stew

Preparation Time: 20 minutes
Cooking Time: 10 minutes
Servings: 4
Ingredients:

- 2 tablespoons olive oil
- 3 cups vegetable broth
- 2 tablespoons lemon juice, fresh
- ½ teaspoon garlic powder
- ½ cup carrots, shredded
- 2 cups cabbage, shredded
- 1 cup beets, shredded

Dill for garnish:

- ½ teaspoon onion powder
- Sea salt and black pepper to taste

Directions:

1. Heat oil in a pot, and then saute your vegetables.
2. Pour your broth in, mixing in your seasoning. Simmer until it's cooked through, and then top with dill.

Nutrition:

- Calories: 263
- Carbohydrates: 8 g
- Protein: 20.3 g
- Fat: 24 g

Basil Tomato Soup

Preparation Time: 10 minutes
Cooking Time: 10 minutes
Servings: 6
Ingredients:

- 28 ounces can tomato
- ¼ cup basil pesto
- ¼ teaspoon dried basil leaves
- 1 teaspoon apple cider vinegar
- 2 tablespoons erythritol
- ¼ teaspoon garlic powder
- ½ teaspoon onion powder
- 2 cups water
- 1-½ teaspoons kosher salt

Directions:

1. Add tomatoes, garlic powder, onion powder, water, and salt to a saucepan.
2. Bring to boil over medium heat. Reduce heat and simmer for 2 minutes.
3. Remove saucepan from heat and puree the soup using a blender until smooth.
4. Stir in pesto, dried basil, vinegar, and erythritol.
5. Stir well and serve warm.

Nutrition:

- Calories: 662
- Carbohydrates: 18 g
- Protein: 8 g
- Fat: 55 g

Broccoli Salad

Preparation Time: 5 minutes
Cooking Time: 25 minutes
Servings: 6
Ingredients:

- 2 tablespoons sherry vinegar
- ¼ cup olive oil
- 2 teaspoons fresh thyme, chopped
- 1 teaspoon Dijon mustard
- 1 teaspoon honey
- Salt to taste
- 8 cups broccoli florets, steamed or roasted
- 2 red onions, sliced thinly
- ½ cup parmesan cheese, shaved
- ¼ cup pecans, toasted and chopped

Directions:

1. Mix the sherry vinegar, olive oil, thyme, mustard, honey and salt in a bowl.
2. In a serving bowl, combine the broccoli florets and onions.
3. Drizzle the dressing on top.
4. Sprinkle with the pecans and parmesan cheese before serving.

Nutrition:

- Calories: 199
- Fat: 17.4 g
- Saturated fat 2.9 g

- Carbohydrates: 7.5 g
- Fiber 2.8 g
- Protein: 5.2 g

Pea Salad

Preparation Time: 40 minutes
Cooking Time: 0 minutes
Servings: 6
Ingredients:
- 1 cup chickpeas, rinsed and drained
- 1-½ cups peas, divided
- Salt to taste
- 3 tablespoons olive oil
- ½ cup buttermilk
- Pepper to taste
- 8 cups pea greens
- 3 carrots, shaved
- 1 cup snow peas, trimmed

Directions:
1. Add the chickpeas and half of the peas to your food processor.
2. Season with salt.
3. Pulse until smooth. Set aside.
4. In a bowl, toss the remaining peas in oil, milk, salt and pepper.
5. Transfer the mixture to your food processor.
6. Process until pureed.
7. Transfer this blend to a bowl.
8. Arrange the pea greens on a serving plate.
9. Top with the shaved carrots and snow peas.
10. Stir in the pea and milk dressing.
11. Serve with the reserved chickpea hummus.

Nutrition:
- Calories: 214
- Fat: 8.6 g
- Saturated fat 1.5 g
- Carbohydrates: 27.3 g
- Fiber 8.4 g
- Protein: 8 g

Snap Pea Salad

Preparation Time: 1 hour
Cooking Time: 0 minutes
Servings: 6
Ingredients:
- 2 tablespoons mayonnaise
- ¾ teaspoon celery seed
- ¼ cup cider vinegar
- 1 teaspoon yellow mustard
- 1 tablespoon sugar
- Salt and pepper to taste
- 4 ounces radishes, sliced thinly
- 12 ounces sugar snap peas, sliced thinly

Directions:
1. In a bowl, combine the mayonnaise, celery seeds, vinegar, mustard, sugar, salt and pepper.
2. Stir in the radishes and snap peas.
3. Refrigerate for 30 minutes.

Nutrition:
- Calories: 69
- Fat: 3.7 g
- Saturated fat 0.6 g
- Carbohydrates: 7.1 g
- Fiber 1.8 g
- Protein: 2 g

Creamy Cauliflower Pakora Soup

Preparation Time: 20 minutes
Cooking Time: 20 minutes
Servings: 8
Ingredients:
- 1 huge head cauliflower, cut into little florets
- 5 medium potatoes, stripped and diced
- 1 huge onion, diced
- 4 medium carrots, stripped and diced
- 2 celery ribs, diced
- 1 container (32 ounces) vegetable stock
- 1 teaspoon garam masala
- 1 teaspoon garlic powder
- 1 teaspoon ground coriander
- 1 teaspoon ground turmeric
- 1 teaspoon ground cumin
- 1 teaspoon pepper
- 1 teaspoon salt
- ½ teaspoon squashed red pepper chips
- Water or extra vegetable stock enough to cover the vegetables
- New cilantro leaves for toppings
- Lime wedges, discretionary

Directions:
1. In a Dutch stove over medium-high fire, heat the initial 14 elements to the point of boiling.
2. Cook and mix until vegetables are delicate, around 20 minutes. Remove from heat; cool marginally. Procedure in groups in a blender or food processor until smooth.
3. Modify consistency as wanted with water (or extra stock). Sprinkle with new cilantro. Serve hot, with lime wedges whenever wanted.

Stop alternative: Before including cilantro, solidify cooled soup in cooler compartments. To use, in part defrost in cooler medium-term.
Warmth through in a pan, blending every so often and including a little water if too thick. Sprinkle with cilantro. Whenever wanted, present with lime wedges.

Nutrition:
- Calories: 248
- Carbohydrates: 7 g
- Protein: 1 g
- Fat: 19 g

Garden Vegetable and Herb Soup

Preparation Time: 20 minutes
Cooking Time: 30 minutes
Servings: 8
Ingredients:
- 2 tablespoons olive oil
- 2 medium onions, hacked
- 2 huge carrots, cut
- 1-pound red potatoes (around 3 medium), cubed
- 2 cups water
- 1 can (14-½ ounces) diced tomatoes in sauce
- 1-½ cups vegetable soup
- 1-½ teaspoons garlic powder
- 1 teaspoon dried basil
- ½ teaspoon salt
- ½ teaspoon paprika
- ¼ teaspoon dill weed
- ¼ teaspoon pepper
- 1 medium yellow summer squash, split and cut
- 1 medium zucchini, split and cut

Directions:
1. In a huge pan, heat oil over medium warmth. Include onions and carrots; cook and mix until onions are delicate, 4-6 minutes. Add potatoes and cook for 2 minutes. Blend in water, tomatoes, juices, and seasonings.
2. Heat to the point of boiling. Lower heat; stew, revealed, until potatoes and carrots are tender, 9 minutes.
3. Include yellow squash and zucchini; cook until vegetables are tender, 9 minutes longer. Serve or, whenever wanted, puree blend in clusters, including extra stock until desired consistency is accomplished.

Nutrition:
- Calories: 252
- Carbohydrates: 12 g
- Protein: 1 g
- Fat: 11 g

Balsamic Artichokes

Preparation Time: 11 minutes
Cooking Time: 8 minutes
Serving: 4
Ingredients:
- 2 teaspoons balsamic vinegar
- Black pepper and salt to taste
- ¼ cup olive oil
- 1 teaspoon oregano
- 4 big trimmed artichokes
- 2 tablespoons lemon juice
- 2 garlic cloves

Directions:
1. Sprinkle the artichokes with pepper and salt.
2. Brush oil over the artichokes and add lemon juice.
3. Place the artichokes on the Power XL Air Fryer Grill.
4. Set the Power XL Air Fryer Grill at Air Fryer/Grill, timer at 7 minutes at 360°Fahrenheit.
5. Mix garlic, lemon juice, pepper, vinegar, oil in a bowl.
6. Add oregano and salt.
7. Combine well.
8. Serve the artichokes with balsamic vinaigrette.

Serving suggestions: Serve with mint chutney.
Directions and cooking tips: Use fresh balsamic.

Nutrition:
- Calories: 533
- Fat: 29 g
- Carbohydrates: 68 g
- Proteins 19 g

Cheesy Artichokes

Preparation Time: 15 minutes
Cooking Time: 6 minutes
Servings: 5
Ingredients:
- 1 teaspoon onion powder
- ½ cup chicken stock
- 14 ounces artichoke hearts
- 8 ounces mozzarella
- ½ cup mayonnaise
- 8 ounces cream cheese
- 10 ounces spinach
- 3 garlic cloves
- 16 ounces grated parmesan cheese
- ½ cup sour cream

Directions:

1. Mix cream cheese, onion powder, chicken stock, and artichokes in a bowl.
2. Add sour cream, mayonnaise, spinach to the bowl.
3. Transfer the mixture to the Power XL Air Fryer Grill pan.
4. Set the Power XL Air Fryer Grill to Air fryer/Grill.
5. Set timer to 6 minutes at 350°Fahrenheit.
6. Serve immediately.

Serving suggestions: Serve with parmesan and mozzarella.

Directions and cooking tips: Rinse artichokes hearts well.

Nutrition:
- Calories: 379
- Fat: 19 g
- Carbohydrates: 36 g
- Proteins 15 g

Beet Salad with Parsley Dressing

Preparation Time: 15 minutes
Cooking Time: 15 minutes
Serving: 4
Ingredients:
- Black pepper and salt to taste
- 1 garlic clove
- 2 tablespoons balsamic vinegar
- 4 beets
- 2 tablespoons capers
- 1 bunch chopped parsley
- 1 tablespoon olive oil

Directions:
1. Place beets on the Power XL Air Fryer Grill pan.
2. Set the Power XL Air Fryer Grill to the air fry function.
3. Set timer and temperature to 15 minutes and 360°Fahrenheit.
4. In another bowl, mix pepper, garlic, capers, salt, and olive oil. Combine well.
5. Remove the beets from the Power XL Air Fryer Grill and place them on a flat surface.
6. Peel and put it in the salad bowl.
7. Serve with vinegar.

Serving suggestions: Dress with parsley mixture.

Directions and cooking tips: Rinse beets before cooking.

Nutrition:
- Calories: 185
- Fat: 16 g
- Carbohydrates: 11 g
- Proteins 8 g

Blue Cheese Salad and Beets

Preparation Time: 15 minutes
Cooking Time: 15 minutes
Servings: 5
Ingredients:
- 1 tablespoon olive oil
- Black pepper and salt to taste
- 6 beets
- ¼ cup blue cheese

Directions:
1. Set the beets on the Power XL Air Fryer Grill pan.
2. Set the Power XL Air Fryer Grill to the air fry function.
3. Set timer to 15 minutes.
4. Cook at 350°Fahrenheit.
5. Transfer it to a plate.
6. Add pepper, blue cheese, oil, and salt.
7. Serve immediately.

Serving suggestions: Serve with maple syrup.

Directions and cooking tips: Peel beets and cut them into quarters.

Nutrition:
- Calories: 110
- Fat: 11 g
- Carbohydrates: 4 g
- Proteins 5 g

Air Fryer Broccoli Salad

Preparation Time: 15 minutes
Cooking Time: 9 minutes
Serving: 4
Ingredients:
- 6 garlic cloves
- 1 head broccoli (about 2 cups)
- Black pepper and salt to taste
- 1 tablespoon Chinese rice wine vinegar
- 1 tablespoon peanut oil

Directions:
1. Mix oil, salt, broccoli, and pepper.
2. Place the blend on the Power XL Air Fryer Grill pan.
3. Set the Power XL Air Fryer Grill to the Air Fry function.
4. Cook for 9 minutes at 350°Fahrenheit.
5. Place the broccoli in the salad bowl and add peanuts oil, rice vinegar, and garlic.
6. Serve immediately.

Serving suggestions: Toss the broccoli well in rice vinegar.

Directions and cooking tips: Separate the broccoli floret.

Nutrition:
- Calories: 199 Fat: 14 g
- Carbohydrates: 17 g
- Proteins 8 g

Brussels Sprout with Tomatoes Mix

Preparation Time: 10 minutes
Cooking Time: 10 minutes
Servings: 3
Ingredients:
- 6 halved cherry tomatoes
- 1 tablespoon olive oil
- 1 pound Brussel sprouts
- Black pepper and salt to taste
- ¼ cup chopped green onions

Directions:
1. Sprinkle pepper and salt on the Brussels sprout.
2. Place it on the Power XL Air Fryer Grill pan.
3. Set the Power XL Air Fryer Grill to the air fry function.
4. Cook for 10 minutes at 350°Fahrenheit.
5. Place the cooked sprout in a bowl, add pepper, green onion, salt, olive oil, and cherry tomatoes.
6. Combine well and serve immediately.

Serving suggestions: Serve with tomato mix or ketchup.
Directions and cooking tips: Trim the Brussels sprout.

Nutrition:
- Calories: 57
- Fat: 1 g
- Carbohydrates: 12 g
- Proteins 5 g

Cucumber Tomato Chopped Salad

Preparation Time: 15 minutes
Cooking Time: 0 minutes
Servings: 6
Ingredients:
- ½ cup light mayonnaise
- 1 tablespoon lemon juice
- 1 tablespoon fresh dill, chopped
- 1 tablespoon chives, chopped
- ½ cup feta cheese, crumbled
- Salt and pepper to taste
- 1 red onion, chopped
- 1 cucumber, diced
- 1 radish, diced
- 3 tomatoes, diced
- Chives, chopped

Directions:
1. Combine the mayonnaise, lemon juice, fresh dill, chives, feta cheese, salt and pepper in a bowl.

2. Mix well.
3. Stir in the onion, cucumber, radish and tomatoes.
4. Coat evenly.
5. Garnish with the chopped chives.

Nutrition:
- Calories: 187
- Fat: 16.7 g
- Saturated fat 4.1 g
- Carbohydrates: 6.7 g
- Fiber 2 g
- Protein: 3.3 g

Zucchini Pasta Salad

Preparation Time: 4 minutes
Cooking Time: 0 minutes
Servings: 15
Ingredients:
- 5 tablespoons olive oil
- 2 teaspoons Dijon mustard
- 3 tablespoons red-wine vinegar
- 1 garlic clove, grated
- 2 tablespoons fresh oregano, chopped
- 1 shallot, chopped
- ¼ teaspoon red pepper flakes
- 16 ounces zucchini noodles
- ¼ cup Kalamata olives, pitted
- 3 cups cherry tomatoes, sliced in half
- ¾ cup parmesan cheese, shaved

Directions:
1. Mix the olive oil, Dijon mustard, red wine vinegar, garlic, oregano, shallot, and red pepper flakes in a bowl.
2. Stir in the zucchini noodles.
3. Sprinkle on top of the olives, tomatoes, and parmesan cheese.

Nutrition:
- Calories: 299
- Fat: 24.7 g
- Saturated fat 5.1 g
- Carbohydrates: 11.6 g
- Fiber 2.8 g
- Protein: 7 g

Egg Avocado Salad

Preparation Time: 10 minutes
Cooking Time: 0 minutes
Servings: 4
Ingredients:
- 1 avocado
- 6 hard-boiled eggs, peeled and chopped
- 1 tablespoon mayonnaise

- 2 tablespoons freshly squeezed lemon juice
- ¼ cup celery, chopped
- 2 tablespoons chives, chopped
- Salt and pepper to taste

Directions:
1. Add the avocado to a large bowl.
2. Mash the avocado using a fork.
3. Stir in the egg and mash the eggs.
4. Add the mayonnaise, lemon juice, celery, chives, salt and pepper.
5. Chill in the refrigerator for at least 28 minutes before serving.

Nutrition:
- Calories: 224
- Fat: 18 g
- Saturated fat 3.9 g
- Carbohydrates: 6.1 g
- Fiber 3.6 g
- Protein: 10.6 g

Arugula Salad

Preparation Time: 15 minutes
Cooking Time: 0 minutes
Servings: 4
Ingredients:
- 6 cups fresh arugula leaves
- 2 cups radicchio, chopped
- ¼ cup low-fat balsamic vinaigrette
- ¼ cup pine nuts, toasted and chopped

Directions:
1. Arrange the arugula leaves in a serving bowl.
2. Sprinkle the radicchio on top.
3. Drizzle with the vinaigrette.
4. Sprinkle the pine nuts on top.
5. Serve

Nutrition:
- Calories: 85
- Fat: 6.6 g
- Saturated fat 0.5 g
- Carbohydrates: 5.1 g
- Fiber 1 g
- Protein: 2.2 g

Mediterranean Salad

Preparation Time: 20 minutes
Cooking Time: 5 minutes
Servings: 2
Ingredients:
- 2 teaspoons balsamic vinegar
- 1 tablespoon basil pesto
- 1 cup lettuce

- ¼ cup broccoli florets, chopped
- ½ cup zucchini, chopped
- ¼ cup tomato, chopped
- ¼ cup yellow bell pepper, chopped
- 2 tablespoons feta cheese, crumbled

Directions:
1. Arrange the lettuce on a serving platter.
2. Top with broccoli, zucchini, tomato and bell pepper.
3. In a bowl, mix the vinegar and pesto.
4. Drizzle the dressing on top.
5. Sprinkle the feta cheese and serve.

Nutrition:
- Calories: 100
- Fat: 6 g
- Saturated fat 1 g
- Carbohydrates: 7 g
- Protein: 4 g

Potato Tuna Salad

Preparation Time: 4 hours and 20 minutes
Cooking Time: 10 minutes
Servings: 6
Ingredients:
- Water enough to cover potatoes
- 3 potatoes, peeled and sliced into cubes
- ½ cup plain yogurt
- ½ cup mayonnaise
- 1 garlic clove, crushed and minced
- 1 tablespoon almond milk
- 1 tablespoon fresh dill, chopped
- ½ teaspoon lemon zest
- Salt to taste
- 1 cup cucumber, chopped
- ¼ cup scallions, chopped
- ¼ cup radishes, chopped
- 9 ounces canned tuna flakes
- 2 hard-boiled eggs, chopped
- 6 cups lettuce, chopped

Directions:
1. Fill your pot with water.
2. Add the potatoes and boil.
3. Cook for 10 minutes or until slightly tender.
4. Drain and let cool.
5. In a bowl, mix the yogurt, mayonnaise, garlic, almond milk, fresh dill, lemon zest and salt.
6. Stir in the potatoes, tuna flakes and eggs.
7. Combine well.
8. Chill in the refrigerator for 4 hours.
9. Stir in the shredded lettuce before serving.

Nutrition:

- Calories: 243 Fat: 9.9 g
- Saturated fat 2 g Carbohydrates: 22.2 g
- Fiber 4.6 g Protein: 17.5 g

Pumpkin Quesadillas

Preparation Time: 10 minutes
Cooking Time: 5 minutes
Servings: 3
Ingredients:
- ½ canned pumpkin (pure)
- 2 gluten-free tortillas
- ½ cup refried beans
- 1-2 tablespoons nutritional yeast
- 1 teaspoon onion powder
- 1 teaspoon garlic powder
- A pinch cayenne
- Salt and pepper to taste

Directions:
1. Mix the pumpkin with nutritional yeast, onion powder, garlic powder, cayenne, salt, and pepper.
2. Spread the pumpkin paste blend in one tortilla and the refried beans in another.
3. Sandwich them together and toast in the Power XL Air Fryer Grill for 5 minutes.
4. Serve

Nutrition:
- Calories: 282
- Carbohydrates: 37 g
- Protein: 13 g
- Fat: 10 g

Brussel Sprouts, Mango, Avocado Salsa Tacos

Preparation Time: 25 minutes
Cooking Time: 15 minutes
Servings: 4
Ingredients:
- 4 taco shells
- 8 ounces Brussels sprouts, diced
- ½ mango, diced
- ½ an avocado, diced
- ½ cup black beans, cooked
- 2 tablespoon onions, chopped
- ¼ cup cilantro, chopped
- 1 tablespoon jalapeno, chopped
- Juice of 1 Lime juice
- 2 Olive oil
- 1 tablespoon taco seasoning

- Salt and pepper to taste

Directions:
1. Preheat the Power XL Air Fryer Grill at 230°Celsius or 400°Fahrenheit.
2. Mix the sprouts with taco seasoning, olive oil, and salt and pepper on the pan.
3. Roast for 15 minutes. Turn every 5 minutes.
4. To make the salsa, combine the mango, avocado, black beans, lime juice, cilantro, onion, jalapeno, salt, and pepper.
5. Cook taco shells and fill them with sprouts and salsa.

Nutrition:
- Calories: 407
- Carbohydrates: 63.20 g
- Protein: 11.4 g
- Fat: 13.9 g

Zucchini Mix and Herbed Eggplant

Preparation Time: 10 minutes
Cooking Time: 8 minutes
Servings: 3
Ingredients:
- 1 teaspoon dried thyme
- 3 tablespoons olive oil
- 1 eggplant
- 2 tablespoons lemon juice
- 1 teaspoon dried oregano
- 3 cubed zucchinis
- Black pepper and salt to taste

Directions:
1. Place the eggplants on the Power XL Air Fryer Grill pan, add thyme, zucchinis, olive oil and salt.
2. Add pepper, oregano, and lemon juice.
3. Set the Power XL Air Fryer Grill to the Air Fry function.
4. Cook for 8 minutes at 360°Fahrenheit.
5. Serve immediately.

Nutrition:
- Calories: 55
- Fat: 1 g
- Carbohydrates: 13 g
- Proteins 3 g

Healthy Mixed Vegetables

Preparation Time: 10 minutes
Cooking Time: 10 minutes
Servings: 6
Ingredients:
- 2 cups mushrooms, cut in half
- 2 yellow squash, sliced
- 2 medium zucchini, sliced

- ¾ teaspoon Italian seasoning
- ½ onion, sliced
- ½ cup olive oil
- ½ teaspoon garlic salt

Directions:
1. Add vegetables and remaining ingredients into the mixing bowl and toss well.
2. Add vegetables into the Air Fryer basket and cook at 400°Fahrenheit for 10 minutes. Shake basket halfway through.
3. Serve and enjoy.

Nutrition:
- Calories: 176
- Fat: 17.3 g
- Carbohydrates: 6.2 g
- Sugar 3.2 g
- Protein: 2.5 g
- Cholesterol 0 mg

African Pineapple Peanut Stew

Preparation Time: 10 minutes
Cooking Time: 20 minutes
Servings: 4
Ingredients:
- 4 cups sliced kale
- 1 cup chopped onion
- ½ cup peanut butter
- 1 tablespoon hot pepper sauce or 1 tablespoon Tabasco sauce
- 2 minced garlic cloves
- ½ cup chopped cilantro
- 2 cups pineapple, undrained, canned and crushed
- 1 tablespoon vegetable oil

Directions:
1. In a saucepan (preferably covered), saute the garlic and onions in the oil until the onions are lightly browned, approximately 10 minutes, stirring often.
2. Wash the kale, till the time the onions are sautéed.
3. Get rid of the stems. Mound the leaves on a cutting surface and slice crosswise into slices (preferably 1 thick).
4. Now put the pineapple and juice to the onions and bring to a simmer. Stir the kale in, cover, and simmer until just tender, stirring frequently for approximately 5 minutes.
5. Mix in the hot pepper sauce, peanut butter and simmer for more than 5 minutes.
6. Add salt according to your taste.

Nutrition:
- Calories: 402
- Carbohydrates: 7 g
- Protein: 21 g
- Fat: 34 g

Amazing Chickpea and Noodle Soup

Preparation Time: 10 minutes
Cooking Time: 20 minutes
Servings: 1 cup
Ingredients:
- 1 freshly diced celery stalk
- ¼ cup chicken seasoning
- 1 cup freshly diced onion
- 3 freshly crushed garlic cloves
- 2 cups cooked chickpeas
- 4 cups vegetable broth
- Freshly chopped cilantro for toppings
- 2 freshly cubed medium-size potatoes
- 2 freshly sliced carrots
- ½ teaspoon dried thyme
- Pepper to taste
- Salt to taste
- 1 cup Water
- 6 ounces gluten-free spaghetti

Directions:
1. Put a pot on medium heat and saute the onion. It will soften within 3 minutes.
2. Add celery, potato, and carrots; then saute for another 3 minutes
3. Add the chicken seasoning to the garlic, thyme, water, and vegetable broth.
4. Simmer the mix on medium-high heat. Cook the veggies for about 20 minutes until they soften.
5. Add the cooked pasta and chickpeas.
6. Add salt and pepper to taste.
7. Put the fresh cilantro on top and enjoy the fresh soup!

Nutrition:
- Calories: 405 Carbohydrates: 1 g
- Protein: 19 g Fat: 38 g

Lentil Soup the Vegan Way

Preparation Time: 5 minutes
Cooking Time: 20 minutes
Servings: 1 cup
Ingredients:
- 2 tablespoons water
- 4 stalks thinly sliced celery
- 2 freshly minced garlic cloves

- 4 thinly sliced large carrots
- Sea salt to taste
- 2 freshly diced small shallots
- Pepper to taste
- 3 cups red/yellow baby potatoes
- 2 cups chopped sturdy greens
- 4 cups vegetable broth
- 1 cup uncooked brown or green lentils
- 1 tbsp Fresh rosemary/thyme

Directions:

1. Put a large pot over medium heat. Once the pot is hot enough, add the shallots, garlic, celery, and carrots to the water. Season the veggies with a little bit of pepper and salt.
2. Saute the veggies for 5 minutes until they are tender. You will know the veggies are ready when they have turned golden brown. Be careful with the garlic because it can easily burn.
3. Add the potatoes and some more seasoning. Cook for 2 minutes.
4. Mix the vegetable broth with the rosemary. Now Increase the heat to medium-high. Allow the veggies to be on a rolling simmer. Add the lentils and give everything a thorough stir.
5. Once it starts to simmer again, decrease the heat and simmer for about 20 minutes without a cover. You will know that veggies are ready when both the lentils and potatoes are soft.
6. Add the greens. Cook for 4 minutes until they wilt. You can adjust the flavor with seasonings.
7. Enjoy this with rice or flatbread. The leftovers are equally tasty. Store them well to enjoy on a day when you are not in the mood to cook.

Nutrition:
- Calories: 284
- Carbohydrates: 21 g
- Protein: 11 g
- Fat: 19 g

Spicy Cabbage

Preparation Time 10 minutes
Cooking Time: 8 minutes
Servings: 5
Ingredients:
- 1 grated carrot
- ½ teaspoon cayenne
- ¼ cup apple cider vinegar
- 1 cabbage
- 1 teaspoon red pepper flakes
- 1 tablespoon sesame seed oil
- ¼ cups apple juice

Directions:

1. Put carrot, cayenne, cabbage, and oil on the Power XL Air Fryer Grill pan.
2. Add vinegar, pepper flakes, and apple juice.
3. Set the Power XL Air Fryer Grill to the air fry function.
4. Cook for 8 minutes at 350°Fahrenheit.
5. Serve immediately

Serving suggestions: Serve with maple syrup.
Directions and cooking tips: Cut the cabbage into 8 wedges.

Nutrition:
- Calories: 25 Fat: 0 g
- Carbohydrates: 6 g
- Proteins 2 g

Sweet Baby Carrots

Preparation Time 15 minutes
Cooking Time: 10 minutes
Serving: 4
Ingredients:
- 1 tablespoon brown sugar
- 2 cups baby carrots
- ½ tablespoon melted butter
- Black pepper and salt

Directions:

1. Mix butter, sugar, pepper, carrot, and salt in a bowl.
2. Transfer the mix to the Power XL Air Fryer Grill pan.
3. Set the Power XL Air Fryer Grill to the air fry function.
4. Cook for 10 minutes at 350°Fahrenheit.
5. Serve immediately.

Serving suggestions: Serve with maple syrup.
Directions and cooking tips: Rinse the carrot before cooking.

Nutrition:
- Calories: 77
- Fat: 3 g
- Carbohydrates: 15 g
- Proteins 3 g

Sweet Potato Toast

Preparation Time: 15 minutes
Cooking Time: 10 minutes
Servings: 2
Ingredients:
- 1 large sweet potato, cut
- 1 Avocado/guacamole
- ¼ cup Hummus
- Radish/Tomato (optional)
- Salt and pepper to taste
- Lemon slice

Directions:

1. Toast the potatoes in the Power XL Air Fryer Grill for 10 minutes on each side.
2. Spread mashed avocado, add seasoning, top it with radish slices and squeeze a lime over it. Or, spread hummus, seasoning, and your choice of greens.

Nutrition:

- Calories: 114
- Carbohydrates: 13 g
- Protein: 2 g
- Fat: 7 g

Spinach Soup with Dill and Basil

Preparation Time: 10 minutes
Cooking Time: 25 minutes
Servings: 8
Ingredients:

- 1 pound peeled and diced potatoes
- 1 tablespoon minced garlic
- 1 teaspoon dry mustard
- 6 cups vegetable broth
- 20 ounces chopped frozen spinach
- 2 cups chopped onion
- 1-½ tablespoons salt
- ½ cup minced dill
- 1 cup basil
- ½ teaspoon ground black pepper

Directions:

1. Whisk onion, garlic, potatoes, broth, mustard, and salt in a pan and cook it over medium flame. When it starts boiling, low down the heat and cover it with the lid and cook for 20 minutes.
2. Add the remaining ingredients in it and blend it then cook it for few more minutes and serve it.

Nutrition:

- Calories: 165
- Carbohydrates: 12 g
- Protein: 13 g
- Fat: 1 g

Chickpea and Spinach Salad

Preparation Time: 5 minutes
Cooking Time: 0 minutes
Servings: 4
Ingredients:

- 2 cans (14-½ ounces each) chickpeas, drained, rinsed
- 7 ounces vegan feta cheese, crumbled or chopped
- 1 tablespoon lemon juice
- ⅓-½ cup olive oil
- ½ teaspoon salt or to taste
- 4-6 cups spinach, torn
- ½ cup raisins
- 2 tablespoons honey
- 1-2 teaspoons ground cumin
- 1 teaspoon chili flakes

Directions:

1. Add cheese, chickpeas, and spinach into a large bowl.

To make the dressing:

1. Add the rest of the ingredients into another bowl and mix well.
2. Pour dressing over the salad. Toss well and serve.

Nutrition:

- Calories: 822
- Fat: 42.5 g
- Saturated fat 11.7 g
- Cholesterol 44 mg
- Sodium 910 mg
- Carbohydrate 89.6 g
- Fiber 19.7 g
- Sugar 32.7 g
- Protein: 29 g
- Vitamin D 0 mcg
- Calcium 417 mg
- Iron 9 mg
- Potassium 1347 mg

Avocado Cucumber Soup

Preparation Time: 20 minutes
Cooking Time: 0 minutes
Servings: 3
Ingredients:

- 1 large cucumber, peeled and sliced
- ¾ cup water
- ¼ cup lemon juice
- 2 garlic cloves
- 6 green onions
- 2 avocados, pitted
- ½ teaspoon black pepper
- ½ teaspoon pink salt

Directions:

1. Add all ingredients into the blender and mixture until smooth and creamy.
2. Place in refrigerator for 30 minutes.
3. Stir well and serve chilled.

Nutrition:

- Calories: 127 Fat: 6.6 g
- Carbohydrates: 13 g

- Protein: 0.7 g

Chapter 4:   Lunch Dishes

Tangy Broccoli Salad

Preparation Time: 15 minutes
Cooking Time: 0 minutes
Servings: 4
Ingredients:

- 2 heads broccoli, stems, and florets chopped (about 5 cups)
- 3 scallions, thinly sliced
- ½ cup carrots, grated
- ¼ cup hemp hearts
- 2 tablespoons tahini
- 2 tablespoons apple cider vinegar
- 2 tablespoons water
- 2 teaspoons maple syrup
- 1 garlic clove
- ¼ teaspoon salt
- Freshly ground black pepper, to taste

Directions:

1. Place the broccoli, scallions, carrots, and hemp hearts in a large bowl. Whisk the tahini, vinegar, water, maple syrup, garlic, and salt in a measuring cup or small bowl. Add as much pepper as you'd like.
2. Put the dressing over the salad and mix until everything is well combined.

Nutrition:

- Calories: 189
- Fat: 11 g
- Carbohydrates: 15 g
- Protein: 10 g

Summer Rolls with Peanut Sauce

Preparation Time: 15 minutes
Cooking Time: 0 minutes
Servings: 4-6
Ingredients:

- 6 to 8 Vietnamese/Thai round rice paper wraps
- 1 (13 ounces) package organic, extra-firm smoked or plain tofu, drained, cut into long, thin slices
- 1 cucumber, cored, cut into matchsticks (about 1 cup)
- 1 cup carrot, cut into matchsticks
- 1 cup mung bean or soybean sprouts
- 4 to 6 cups spinach
- 12 to 16 basil leaves
- 3 to 4 mint sprigs
- Sweet peanut dressing

Directions:

1. Place the rice paper wrap under running water or in a large bowl of water for a moment, then set it on a plate or cutting board to absorb the water for 30 seconds. The wrap should be transparent and pliable.
2. Place your desired amount of filling on each wrap, being careful not to overfill because they will be hard to close.
3. Tightly fold the bottom of the wraps over the ingredients, and then fold in each side. Continue rolling each wrap onto itself to form the rolls. Enjoy your rolls dipped in sweet peanut dressing.

Nutrition:

- Calories: 216
- Fat: 6 g
- Carbohydrates: 32 g
- Protein: 13 g

Vegetable Rose Potato

Preparation Time: 15 minutes
Cooking Time: 20 minutes
Servings: 4
Ingredients:

- 4 red rose potatoes
- 6 leaves Lacinato kale, stemmed, chopped
- 2 tablespoons olive oil
- 1 onion, chopped
- 1 green bell pepper, diced
- Ground pepper and salt, to taste

Directions:

1. Microwave your potatoes until done but still firm. Finely chop them when cool.
2. Preheat oil in a skillet over medium heat. Saute onions until translucent. Add potatoes and bell pepper and saute, stirring constantly, over medium-high heat until golden brown.
3. Stir in the kale and seasoning, then cook, stirring constantly until the mixture is a bit browned. Occasionally add water to prevent sticking if necessary. Sprinkle with pepper and salt to taste. Serve hot.
4.

Nutrition:

- Calories: 337 Fat: 7.4 g

- Carbohydrates: 63 g Protein: 8 g

Tomato Salad

Preparation Time: 15 minutes
Cooking Time: 0 minutes
Servings: 4
Ingredients:

- 1 head romaine lettuce, washed, chopped
- 1 avocado, sliced
- 24 cherry tomatoes
- ½ cup cilantro, chopped
- Fresh lime juice, for dressing

Directions:

1. Divide all the ingredients between 4 plates and drizzle with lime juice dressing.
2. Toss well to combine.
3. Enjoy immediately.

Nutrition:

- Calories: 203 Fat: 16.2 g
- Carbohydrates: 12 g
- Protein: 6 g

Garden Pasta Salad

Preparation Time: 10 minutes
Cooking Time: 12 minutes
Servings: 4
Ingredients:
For the Salad:

- 1 cup chopped kale
- ¼ cup chopped basil
- 2 cups sliced yellow cherry tomatoes
- 16 ounces tri-colored pasta

For the Dressing:

- ½ teaspoon sea salt
- ¼ teaspoon ground black pepper
- 1 teaspoon dried Italian seasoning
- ½ cup white wine vinegar
- 3 tablespoons lemon juice
- 1 teaspoon olive oil

Directions:

1. Cook the pasta. For this, take a large pot half full with salty water, place it over medium heat and bring it to a boil.
2. Add pasta, cook within 10 to 12 minutes until tender, and then drain well into a colander.
3. While pasta cooks, prepare the dressing. For this, take a small bowl, place all of its ingredients in it and whisk until combined.
4. Transfer pasta into a large bowl. Add remaining ingredients for the salad; drizzle with prepared dressing and then toss until well combined.
5. Serve straight away.

Nutrition:

- Calories: 424 Fat: 3 g
- Carbohydrates: 46 g
- Protein: 13 g

Apple Spinach Salad

Preparation Time: 15 minutes
Cooking Time: 0 minutes
Servings: 4
Ingredients:

- 5 ounces fresh spinach
- ¼ red onion, sliced
- 1 apple, sliced
- ¼ cup sliced toasted almonds

For the Dressing:

- 3 tablespoons red wine vinegar
- ⅓ cup olive oil
- 1 minced garlic clove
- 2 teaspoons Dijon mustard
- Salt and pepper, to taste

Directions:

1. Combine red wine vinegar, olive oil, garlic, and Dijon mustard in a bowl. Season with black pepper and salt.
2. In a separate bowl mix fresh spinach, apple, onion, toasted almonds. Pour the dressing on top and toss to combine. Serve

Nutrition:

- Calories: 232
- Fat: 20.8 g
- Carbohydrates: 10 g
- Protein: 3 g

Falafel Kale Salad with Tahini Dressing

Preparation Time: 15 minutes
Cooking Time: 0 minutes
Servings: 4
Ingredients:

- 12 balls Vegan Falafels
- 6 cups kale, chopped
- ½ red onion, thinly sliced
- 2 slices pita bread, cut into squares
- 1 jalapeno, chopped

Tahini Dressing:

- 1-2 lemons, juiced

Directions:

1. In a mixing bowl, combine kale and lemon juice and toss well to mix. Place into the refrigerator. Divide kale among four bowls.
2. Top with three Falafel balls, red onion, jalapeno and pita slices. Top with tahini dressing and serve.

Nutrition:
- Calories: 178
- Fat: 2.8 g
- Carbohydrates: 16 g
- Protein: 4 g

Fig and Kale Salad

Preparation Time: 15 minutes
Cooking Time: 0 minutes
Servings: 2
Ingredients:
- 1 ripe avocado
- 2 tablespoons lemon juice
- 3-½ ounces kale, packed, stems removed, and cut into large-sized bits
- 1 carrot, shredded
- 1 yellow zucchini, diced
- 4 fresh figs
- ¼ cup ground flaxseed
- 1 cup mixed green leaves
- 1 teaspoon sea salt

Directions:
1. Add kale to a bowl with avocado, lemon juice and sea salt.
2. Massage together until kale wilts.
3. Add in zucchini, carrot, and 2 cups mixed green leaves.
4. Fold in figs and remaining ingredients.
5. Toss and serve.

Nutrition:
- Calories: 255
- Fat: 12.5 g
- Carbohydrates: 35 g
- Protein: 6 g

Cucumber Avocado Toast

Preparation Time: 15 minutes
Cooking Time: 0 minutes
Servings: 2
Ingredients:
- 1 cucumber, sliced
- 2 sprouted (Essene) bread slices, toasted
- ¼ handful basil leaves, chopped
- 4 tablespoons avocado, mashed
- Salt and pepper, to taste
- 1 teaspoon lemon juice

Directions:
1. Combine lemon juice together with the mashed avocado, and then spread the mixture on two bread slices.

Top with cucumber slices along with the finely chopped basil leaves. Generously sprinkle with salt and pepper.
2. Enjoy!

Nutrition:
- Calories: 232
- Fat: 14 g
- Carbohydrates: 24 g
- Protein: 5 g

Kale and Cucumber Salad

Preparation Time: 15 minutes
Cooking Time: 50 minutes
Servings: 2
Ingredients:
- 1 garlic clove
- 3-½ ounces fresh ginger
- ½ green Thai chili
- 1-½ tablespoons sugar
- 1-½ tablespoons fish sauce
- 1-½ tablespoons vegetable oil
- 1 English cucumber, thinly sliced
- 1 bunch red Russian kale, ribs and stems removed; leaves torn into small pieces
- 1 Persian cucumber, thinly sliced
- 2 tablespoons fresh lime juice
- 1 small red onion, sliced
- 1 teaspoon sugar
- 2 tablespoons cilantro, chopped
- Salt, to taste

Directions:
1. Heat the broiler and broil ginger, with skin for 50 minutes, turning once. Let cool and slice. Blend chili, ginger, garlic, sugar, fish sauce, oil, and 2 tablespoons of water in a blender until paste forms.
2. Toss ¼ cup of dressing and kale in a bowl and coat well. Massage with hands until kale softens.
3. Toss Persian and English cucumbers, lime juice, onion, and sugar in a bowl; then season with salt. Let it sit for 10 minutes.
4. Add the cucumber mixture to the bowl with kale and toss to combine.
5. Top with cilantro and serve.

Nutrition:
- Calories: 160 Fat: 8 g
- Carbohydrates: 22 g Protein: 3 g

Mexican Quinoa

Preparation Time: 15 minutes
Cooking Time: 8 minutes
Servings: 4

Ingredients:
- 1 cup quinoa, uncooked and rinsed
- 1-½ cups vegetable broth
- 3 cups diced tomatoes
- 2 cups frozen corn
- 1 cup fresh parsley, chopped
- 1 onion, chopped
- 3 garlic cloves, minced
- 2 bell peppers, chopped
- 1 tablespoon paprika powder
- ½ tablespoon cumin
- 2 tablespoons olive oil
- 2 tablespoons lime juice
- 2 green onions, chopped
- Salt and pepper, to taste

Directions:
1. Place a large pot over medium heat. Add olive oil. Cook onions for 3 minutes. Add garlic, bell peppers and cook for 5 minutes.
2. Add the remaining ingredients except for lime juice, green onions and parsley. Cover and cook for about 20 minutes. Keep checking to make sure the quinoa doesn't stick and burn.
3. Add lime juice, green onions and parsley.
4. Season the food with salt and pepper before serving.

Nutrition:
- Calories: 231
- Fat: 17.8 g
- Carbohydrates: 19 g
- Protein: 2 g

Mediterranean Parsley Salad

Preparation Time: 15 minutes
Cooking Time: 0 minutes
Servings: 2
Ingredients:
- ½ red onion, thinly sliced
- 1 cup parsley, chopped
- 1 Roma tomato, seeded and diced
- 6 mints, chopped
- 3 tablespoons currants, died
- 1 green chili, minced
- 1 tablespoon lemon juice
- 2 tablespoons olive oil
- ⅛ teaspoon sumac
- ⅛ teaspoon pepper, cracked
- ¼ teaspoon salt

Directions:
1. Mix lemon juice, olive oil, sumac, salt, and pepper in a bowl and whisk to combine well.

Toss parsley with the remaining ingredients in a separate bowl.
Add the olive oil mixture to it and toss well and serve.

Nutrition:
- Calories: 110
- Fat: 8 g
- Carbohydrates: 7 g
- Protein: 1 g

Tomatoes Parsley Salad

Preparation Time: 15 minutes
Cooking Time: 0 minutes
Servings: 2
Ingredients:
- 2 cups curly parsley leaves, packed
- ¾ cup oil-packed sundried tomatoes, drained and julienned
- 2 tablespoons olive oil
- ½ cup basil leaves
- 2 tablespoons rice vinegar
- 1 shallot, minced
- 1 garlic clove, minced
- Salt and black pepper, to taste

Directions:
1. Wash parsley, dry, and add to a bowl. Add garlic and tomatoes. Toss well. Wash basil and dry it. Add it to a blender and add vinegar, oil, salt, and pepper to it. Mixture until smooth.
2. Add garlic and shallots to the dressing. Add the dressing over the salad and toss well.
3. Divide among 6 salad plates and serve.

Nutrition:
- Calories: 245
- Fat: 19.8 g
- Carbohydrates: 12 g
- Protein: 7 g

Slow Cooker Chili

Preparation Time: 15 minutes
Cooking Time: 9 hours
Servings: 12
Ingredients:
- 3 cups dry pinto beans
- 1 large onion, chopped
- 3 bell peppers, chopped
- 8 large green jalapeno peppers, dice after removing seeds by scraping out
- 2x14-½ ounces cans diced tomatoes, or equivalent
- 1 tablespoon chili powder
- 2 tablespoons oregano flakes
- 1 tablespoon cumin powder

- 1 tablespoon garlic powder
- 3 bay leaves, freshly ground
- 1 teaspoon ground black pepper
- 1 tablespoon sea salt (or to taste)
- Water enough to cover

Directions:
1. Put the beans into your large pan, filled with water, and leave to soak overnight. The next morning, drain and transfer to a 6-quart slow cooker.
2. Cover with salt and two inches of water. Cook on high for 6 hours until soft. Drain the beans and add the other ingredients. Stir well to combine. Cover and cook again within 3 hours on high.
3. Serve and enjoy.

Nutrition:
- Calories: 216 Carbohydrates: 30 g
- Fat: 1 g Protein: 12 g

Spicy Hummus Quesadillas

Preparation Time: 5 minutes
Cooking Time: 15 minutes
Servings: 4
Ingredients:
- 4x8 whole-grain tortilla
- 1 cup hummus

Your choice of fillings:
- Spinach, sundried tomatoes, olives, etc.
- Extra-virgin olive oil for brushing

To serve:
- Extra hummus
- Hot sauce
- Pesto

Directions:
1. Put your tortillas on a flat surface and cover each with hummus. Add the fillings, then fold over to form a half-moon shape.
2. Pop a skillet over medium heat and add a drop of oil. Add the quesadillas and flip when browned. Repeat with the remaining quesadillas; then serve and enjoy.

Nutrition:
- Calories: 256
- Carbohydrates: 25 g
- Fat: 12 g
- Protein: 7 g

Crunchy Rainbow Salad

Preparation Time: 15 minutes
Cooking Time: 0 minutes
Servings: 6

Ingredients:
- 4 cups shredded cabbage, red or green, or bagged slaw mix
- 2 cups cooked edamame
- 1 cup grated or shredded carrots
- ½ bunch cilantro, coarsely chopped
- 2 scallions, thinly sliced
- ½ cup dry roasted peanuts, chopped
- ¾ cup sweet peanut dressing
- Salt, to taste

Directions:
1. Combine the cabbage, edamame, carrots, cilantro, scallions, and dry roasted peanuts in a medium bowl and mix well.
2. Add the peanut dressing and blend again, ensuring the dressing is evenly distributed; season with salt to taste.

Nutrition:
- Calories: 276
- Fat: 16 g
- Carbohydrates: 21 g
- Protein: 20 g

Spicy Peanut Bowl

Preparation Time: 25 minutes
Cooking Time: 0 minutes
Servings: 4
Ingredients:
- 1 (8 ounces) package black bean noodles, cooked
- 2 cups cooked edamame beans
- 1 cup red cabbage, thinly sliced
- 1 cup carrots, grated or shredded
- 1 cup red peppers, finely chopped
- 1 cup mung bean or soybean sprouts
- ¼ cup dry roasted peanuts, coarsely chopped
- ¼ cup cilantro, coarsely chopped
- 4 scallions, coarsely chopped
- 2 tbsp Sweet peanut dressing
- Hot sauce or red chili flakes (optional)

Directions:
1. Divide the noodles evenly among 4 food storage containers. Top each container of noodles with ½ cup of edamame, ¼ cup of cabbage, ¼ cup of carrots, ¼ cup of peppers, ¼ cup of sprouts, and 1 tablespoon of peanuts.
2. Garnish each container with cilantro and scallions. Top it with 3 tablespoons of peanut dressing and hot sauce or chili flakes (if using). Cover the remaining containers with airtight lids and store them in the refrigerator.

Nutrition:
- Calories: 417
- Fat: 11 g
- Carbohydrates: 69 g
- Protein: 14 g

Burrito Bowl

Preparation Time: 15 minutes
Cooking Time: 20 minutes
Servings: 4
Ingredients:
- 1 tablespoon olive oil
- 1 red onion, thinly sliced
- 1 bell pepper, thinly sliced
- A pinch salt
- 1 garlic clove, minced
- ½ teaspoon cumin
- 2 cups white or brown rice, cooked
- 1 (14 ounces) can pinto beans, drained and rinsed
- 4 cups spinach or arugula, chopped
- 1 avocado, chopped
- 4 scallions, coarsely chopped
- Hot sauce or salsa
- Cilantro lime dressing

Directions:
1. In a small skillet, warm the oil over medium-high heat. Add the onion, bell pepper, and a big pinch of salt. Saute for 15 minutes or until the onions begin to caramelize slightly. Add the garlic and cumin and cook for 3 more minutes. Set aside.
2. Set out 4 food storage containers. To each container, add ½ cup of rice, ¼ of the bell pepper mixture, ¼ cup of beans, 1 cup of greens, and ¼ of the avocado.
3. Garnish each container with scallions and a hot sauce or salsa of your choice.

Nutrition:
- Calories: 483
- Fat: 31 g
- Carbohydrates: 50 g
- Protein: 10 g
-

Farro with Pistachios & Herbs

Preparation Time: 20 minutes
Cooking Time: 45 minutes
Servings: 10
Ingredients:
- 2 cups farro
- 4 cups water

- 1 teaspoon kosher salt, divided
- 2-½ tablespoons extra-virgin olive oil
- 1 onion, chopped
- 2 garlic cloves, minced
- ½ teaspoon ground pepper, divided
- ½ cup parsley, chopped
- 4 ounces salted shelled pistachios, toasted, chopped

Directions:
1. Combine farro, water, and ¾ teaspoon salt, simmer for 40 minutes. Cook onion plus garlic in 2 tablespoon oil for 5 minutes.
2. Combine ½ teaspoon oil, ¼ teaspoon pepper, parsley, pistachios, and toss well. Combine all. Season with salt and pepper.

Nutrition:
- Calories: 220
- Carbohydrates: 30 g
- Fat: 9 g
- Protein: 8 g

Stuffed Peppers

Preparation Time: 15 minutes
Cooking Time: 15 minutes
Servings: 8
Ingredients:
- 2 cans black beans, (15 ounces), drained and rinsed
- 2 cups tofu, pressed, crumbled
- ¾ cup green onion s, thinly sliced
- ½ cup fresh cilantro, chopped
- ¼ cup vegetable oil
- ¼ cup lime juice
- 3 garlic cloves, finely chopped
- ½ teaspoon salt
- ½ teaspoon chili powder
- 8 large bell peppers, halved lengthwise, deseeded
- 3 Roma tomatoes, diced

Directions:
1. Mix in a bowl all the fixings except the bell peppers to make the filling. Fill the peppers with this mixture.
2. Cut 8 aluminum foils of size 18 x 12 inches. Place 2 halves on each aluminum foil. Seal the peppers such that there is a gap on the sides.
3. Grill under direct heat within 15 minutes. Sprinkle with some cilantro and serve.

Nutrition:
- Calories: 243
- Carbohydrates: 28 g
- Fat: 7 g

- Protein: 19 g

Sweet and Spicy Tofu

Preparation Time: 15 minutes
Cooking Time: 30 minutes
Servings: 8
Ingredients:

- 14 ounces extra-firm tofu; press the excess liquid and chop into cubes
- 3 tablespoons olive oil
- 2-3 garlic cloves, minced
- 4 tablespoons sriracha sauce or any other hot sauce
- 2 tablespoons soy sauce
- ¼ cup sweet chili sauce
- 5-6 cups mixed vegetables your choice (like carrots, cauliflower, broccoli, potato, etc.)
- Salt to taste (optional)

Directions:

1. Place a non-stick pan over medium-high heat. Add 1 tablespoon of oil. When oil is hot, add garlic and mixed vegetables and stir-fry until crisp and tender. Remove and keep aside.
2. Place the pan back on the heat. Add 2 tablespoons of oil. When oil is hot, add tofu and saute until golden brown. Add the sautéed vegetables. Mix well and remove from heat.
3. Make a mixture of sauces by mixing together all the sauces in a small bowl. Serve the stir-fried vegetables and tofu with sauce.

Nutrition:

- Calories: 270
- Carbohydrates: 41 g
- Fat: 10 g
- Protein: 12 g

Yucatan Bean & Pumpkin Seed

Preparation Time: 10 minutes
Cooking Time: 3 minutes
Servings: 8
Ingredients:

- ¼ cup pumpkin seeds
- 1 can white beans
- 1 tomato, chopped
- ⅓ cup onion, chopped
- ⅓ cup cilantro, chopped
- 4 tablespoons lime juice
- Salt and pepper, to taste

Directions:

1. Toast the pumpkin seeds for 3 minutes to lightly brown.

2. Let cool, and then chop in a food processor.
3. Mix in the remaining ingredients.
4. Season with salt and pepper, then serve.

Nutrition:

- Calories: 12 Fat: 2 g
- Carbohydrates: 12 g
- Protein: 5 g

Corn and Potato Chowder

Preparation Time: 5 minutes
Cooking Time: 35 minutes
Servings: 4
Ingredients:

- 2 ears corn
- 10 ounces tofu, extra-firm, drained cubed
- 1-½ cups frozen corn kernels
- ¼ medium onion, peeled, chopped
- 3 medium potatoes, peeled, cubed
- ¼ medium red bell pepper, cored, chopped
- ¼ cup cilantro, chopped
- ⅔ teaspoon salt
- ¼ cup coconut cream
- 7 cups vegetable broth

Directions:

1. Prepare the ears of corn. For this, remove their skin and husk; then cut each corn into four pieces and place them in a large pot.
2. Place the pot over medium-high heat. Add cilantro, onion, and bell pepper; pour in the broth and bring the mixture to boil. Then switch heat to medium level and cook for 20 minutes until corn pieces are tender.
3. Add potatoes. Cook for 8 minutes until fork tender. Then add tofu and kernels. Simmer for 5 minutes and taste to adjust seasoning.
4. Remove pot from heat, stir in cream until combined and serve straight away.

Nutrition:

- Calories: 159
- Fat: 2.4 g
- Carbohydrates: 29 g
- Protein: 6.6 g

Cauliflower Soup

Preparation Time: 10 minutes
Cooking Time: 40 minutes
Servings: 2
Ingredients:

- 1 small head cauliflower, sliced into florets
- 4 tablespoons pomegranate seeds

- 2 sprigs thyme and more for garnishing
- 1 teaspoon minced garlic
- $^2/_3$ teaspoon salt
- $^1/_3$ teaspoon ground black pepper
- 1 tablespoon olive oil
- 1-½ cups vegetable stock
- ½ cup coconut milk, unsweetened

Directions:

1. Take a pot and place it over medium heat. Add oil and when hot, add garlic and cook for 1 minute until fragrant. Add florets, thyme, pour in the stock, and bring the mixture to boil.

2. Switch heat to the medium low level, simmer the soup for 30 minutes until florets are tender. Then remove the pot from heat, discard the thyme, and puree using an immersion blender until smooth.

3. Stir milk into the soup and season with salt and black pepper. Then garnish with pomegranate seeds and thyme sprigs and serve.

Nutrition:

- Calories: 184
- Fat: 11 g
- Carbohydrates: 17 g
- Protein: 3 g

Chapter 5:   Dinner

Eggplant and Mushrooms in Peanut Sauce

Preparation Time: 15 minutes
Cooking Time: 25 minutes
Servings: 6
Ingredients:

- 4 Japanese eggplants cut into 1-inch-thick round slices
- ¾ pounds shiitake mushrooms, stems discarded, halved
- 3 tablespoons smooth peanut butter
- 2-½ tablespoons rice vinegar
- 1-½ tablespoons soy sauce
- 1-½ tablespoons, peeled, fresh ginger, finely grated
- 1-½ tablespoons light brown sugar
- Coarse salt to taste
- 3 scallions, cut into 2-inch lengths, thinly sliced lengthwise

Directions:

1. Place the eggplants and mushrooms in a steamer. Steam the eggplant and mushrooms until tender. Transfer to a bowl. Put peanut butter and vinegar into a small bowl, and whisk.
2. Add the rest of the fixings and whisk well. Add this to the bowl of eggplant slices. Add scallions and combine well. Serve hot.

Nutrition:

- Calories: 104
- Carbohydrates: 11 g
- Fat: 6 g
- Protein: 4 g

Dijon Maple Burgers

Preparation Time: 20 minutes
Cooking Time: 30 minutes
Servings: 12
Ingredients:

- 1 red bell pepper
- 19 ounces can chickpeas, rinsed and drained
- 1 cup almonds, ground
- 2 teaspoons Dijon mustard
- 1 teaspoon oregano
- ½ teaspoon sage
- 1 cup spinach, fresh

- 1-½ cups rolled oats
- 1 garlic clove, pressed
- ½ lemon, juiced
- 2 teaspoons maple syrup, pure

Directions:

1. Get out a baking sheet. Line it with parchment paper. Cut your red pepper in half and then take the seeds out. Place it on your baking sheet, and roast in the oven while you prepare your other ingredients.
2. Process your chickpeas, almonds, mustard, and maple syrup together in a food processor. Add in your lemon juice, oregano, sage, garlic, and spinach, processing again. Make sure it's combined, but don't puree it.
3. Once your red bell pepper is softened, which should roughly take ten minutes. Add this to the processor as well. Add in your oats, mixing well.
4. Form twelve patties, cooking in the oven for a half-hour. They should be browned.

Nutrition:

- Calories: 96
- Protein: 5.28 g
- Fat: 2.42 g
- Carbohydrates: 16.82 g

Chickpea Salad Bites

Preparation Time: 15 minutes
Cooking Time: 0 minutes
Servings: 4
Ingredients:
For the Bread:

- 2 tablespoons chopped parsley
- 1 small green chili pepper
- ⅓ cup raisins
- 1 teaspoon garlic powder
- ½ teaspoon salt
- ⅓ teaspoon ground black pepper
- ½ teaspoon smoked paprika
- ½ tablespoon maple syrup
- ½ teaspoon cayenne pepper
- 2 tablespoons balsamic vinegar
- 1-½ cups crumbled rye bread, whole-grain

For the Salad:

- 2 scallions, chopped
- ⅓ cup chopped pickles

- 2 tablespoons chopped chives and more for topping
- ½ teaspoon minced garlic
- 1-½ cups cooked chickpeas
- 1 lemon, juiced
- ½ teaspoon salt
- ¼ teaspoon ground black pepper
- 1 tablespoon poppy seed
- 1 teaspoon mustard paste
- ⅓ cup coconut yogurt

Directions:
1. Prepare the bread. For this, place all of its ingredients in a food processor and then pulse for 1 minute until just combined; don't overmix.
2. Then make bites of the bread mixture. For this, take a 2.3-inch round cookie cutter and add 2 tablespoons of the bread mixture. Press it into the cutter and gently lift it out; repeat with the remaining batter to make seven more bites.
3. Prepare the salad. For this, take a large bowl and add chickpeas in it. Then add chives, scallion, pickles, and garlic. Next, mash chickpeas by using a fork until broken.
4. Add remaining ingredients for the salad and stir until well mixed. Assemble the bites. For this, top each prepared bread bite generously with prepared salad. Sprinkle with chives and poppy seeds, and then serve.

Nutrition:
- Calories: 210
- Fat: 4 g
- Carbohydrates: 36 g
- Protein: 7 g

Avocado and Chickpeas Lettuce Cups

Preparation Time: 10 minutes
Cooking Time: 0 minutes
Servings: 4
Ingredients:
- 2 small avocados, peeled, pitted, diced
- 8 ounces hearts palm
- ¾ cup cooked chickpeas
- ½ cup cucumber, diced
- 1 tablespoon minced shallots
- 2 cups mixed greens
- 1 tablespoon Dijon mustard
- 1 lime, zested, juiced
- 2 tablespoons chopped cilantro and more for topping
- ⅔ teaspoon salt
- ⅓ teaspoon ground black pepper
- 1 tablespoon apple cider vinegar
- 2-½ tablespoons olive oil

Directions:
1. Take a medium bowl, add shallots and cilantro in it. Stir in salt, black pepper, mustard, vinegar, lime juice, and zest until just mixed, and then slowly mix in olive oil until combined.
2. Add cucumber, hearts of palm, and chickpeas. Stir until mixed; fold in avocado and then top with some more cilantro.
3. Distribute mixed greens among four plates. Top with chickpea mixture; then serve.

Nutrition:
- Calories: 280
- Fat: 12.6 g
- Carbohydrates: 32.8 g
- Protein: 7.6 g

Pumpkin Risotto

Preparation Time: 5 minutes
Cooking Time: 20 minutes
Servings: 4
Ingredients:
- 1 cup Arborio rice
- ½ cup cooked and chopped pumpkin
- ½ cup mushrooms
- 1 rib celery, diced
- ½ a medium white onion, peeled, diced
- ½ teaspoon minced garlic
- ½ teaspoon salt
- ⅓ teaspoon ground black pepper
- 1 tablespoon olive oil
- ½ tablespoon coconut butter
- 1 cup pumpkin puree
- 2 cups vegetable stock

Directions:
1. Take a medium saucepan, place it over medium heat. Add oil, and when hot, incorporate onion and celery. Stir in garlic, and cook for 3 minutes until onions begin to soften.
2. Put mushrooms, flavor with salt and black pepper. Cook for 5 minutes.
3. Add rice and pour in pumpkin puree. Then gradually pour in the stock until rice soaked up all the liquid and have turned soft.
4. Add butter and remove the pan from heat. Stir until creamy mixture comes together, and then serve.

Nutrition:
- Calories: 218.5
- Fat: 5.2 g

- Carbohydrates: 32.3 g
- Protein: 6.3 g

Chickpea Noodle Soup

Preparation Time: 5 minutes
Cooking Time: 18 minutes
Servings: 6
Ingredients:

- 1 cup cooked chickpeas
- 8 ounces rotini noodles, whole-wheat
- 4 celery stalks, sliced
- 2 medium white onions, peeled, chopped
- 4 medium carrots, peeled, sliced
- 2 teaspoons minced garlic
- 8 sprigs thyme
- 1 teaspoon salt
- $1/3$ teaspoon ground black pepper
- 1 bay leaf
- 2 tablespoons olive oil
- 2 quarts vegetable broth
- $1/4$ cup chopped fresh parsley

Directions:

1. Take a large pot and place it over medium heat. Add oil, and when hot, add all the vegetables. Stir in garlic, thyme, and bay leaf and cook for 5 minutes until vegetables are golden and saute.
2. Then pour in broth stir and bring the mixture to boil. Add chickpeas and noodles into boiling soup. Continue cooking for 8 minutes until noodles are tender. Then season soup with salt and black pepper. Garnish with parsley and serve straight away.

Nutrition:

- Calories: 260
- Fat: 5 g
- Carbohydrates: 44 g
- Protein: 7 g

Red Pepper and Tomato Soup

Preparation Time: 10 minutes
Cooking Time: 40 minutes
Servings: 4
Ingredients:

- 2 carrots, peeled, chopped
- 1-$1/4$ pounds red bell peppers, deseeded, sliced into quarters
- $1/2$ medium red onion, peeled, sliced into thin wedges
- 16 ounces small tomatoes, halved
- 1 tablespoon chopped basil
- $1/2$ teaspoon salt

- 2 cups vegetable broth

Directions:

1. Switch on the oven; then set it to 450°Fahrenheit and let it preheat. Place all the vegetables in a single on a baking sheet lined with foil and roast for 40 minutes until the skins of peppers are slightly charred.
2. When done, remove the baking sheet from the oven and let them cool for 10 minutes. Then peel the peppers and transfer all the vegetables into a blender.
3. Add basil and salt to the vegetables. Pour in the broth and puree the vegetables until smooth. Serve straight away.

Nutrition:

- Calories: 77.4 Fat: 1.8 g
- Carbohydrates: 14.4 g Protein: 3.3 g

Spicy Cilantro and Coconut Soup

Preparation Time: 15 minutes
Cooking Time: 3-5 minutes
Servings: 2
Ingredients:

- 2 tablespoon cilantro leaves
- 1 Jalapeno
- 1 tablespoon lime juice
- 13-$1/2$ ounces full-fat coconut milk
- $1/4$ teaspoon sea salt
- 3 cloves crushed garlic
- $1/4$ cup diced onion
- 2 tablespoons avocado oil

Directions:

1. Add the avocado oil to a medium pan and heat. Add in the salt, garlic, and onion, cooking for 3 to 5 minutes, either that or till the onion bulbs get to be smooth.
2. Put in the onion mixture, cilantro, jalapeno, lime juice, and coconut milk to a blender and mix until it becomes creamy.

3. Pour into a bowl and enjoy.

Nutrition:
- Calories: 114
- Carbohydrates: 14 g
- Fat: 5 g
- Protein: 2 g

Mint and Berry Soup

Preparation Time: 35 minutes
Cooking Time: 30 minutes
Servings: 1
Ingredients:
Sweetener:
- ¼ cup water, plus more if needed
- ¼ cup unrefined whole cane sugar

Soup:
- ½ cup water
- 1 cup mixed berries
- 8 mint leaves
- 1 teaspoon lemon juice

Directions:
1. Put the water and sugar in a small pot and cook, stirring constantly, until the sugar has dissolved. Allow this to cool.
2. Add the mint leaves, lemon juice, water, berries, and the cooled sugar mixture to a blender. Mix everything together until smooth.
3. Pour into a basin then put in the refrigerator till the broth is completely chilled. This will take about 20 minutes. Enjoy.

Nutrition:
- Calories: 240
- Carbohydrates: 14 g
- Fat: 17 g
- Protein: 6 g

Mushroom Soup

Preparation Time: 15 minutes
Cooking Time: 10 minutes
Servings: 2
Ingredients:
- 13-½ ounces full-fat coconut milk
- 1 cup vegetable broth
- ½ teaspoon pepper
- ¾ teaspoon sea salt
- 1 crush garlic clove
- 1 cup diced onion
- 1 cup cut-up Cremini mushrooms
- 1 cup cut-up Chinese black mushrooms
- 1 tablespoon avocado oil
- 1 tablespoon coconut aminos

- ½ teaspoon Dried thyme

Directions:
1. Warm up the grease in a very massive pan and put in all the seasonings: pepper, salt, garlic, onion bulb, and mushrooms.
2. Boil and prepare everything along for a few minutes, either that or till the onions turn soft. Mix in the coconut aminos, thyme, coconut milk, and vegetable broth.
3. Lower the fire down; then allow the broth to boil for approximately a quarter-hour. Mix the broth from time to time. Taste and adjust any of the seasonings you need to. Divide into two bowls and enjoy.

Nutrition:
- Calories: 129
- Carbohydrates: 4 g
- Fat: 10 g
- Protein: 2 g

Pasta with Kidney Bean Sauce

Preparation Time: 5 minutes
Cooking Time: 15 minutes
Servings: 4
Ingredients:
- 12 ounces cooked kidney beans
- 7 ounces whole-wheat pasta, cooked
- 1 medium white onion, peeled, diced
- 1 cup arugula
- 2 tablespoons tomato paste
- 1 teaspoon minced garlic
- ½ teaspoon smoked paprika
- 1 teaspoon dried oregano
- ½ teaspoon cayenne pepper
- ⅓ teaspoon ground black pepper
- ⅔ teaspoon salt
- 2 tablespoons balsamic vinegar

Directions:
1. Take a large skillet pan and place it over medium heat. Add oil, and when hot, add onion and garlic, splash with some water and cook for 5 minutes.
2. Then add remaining ingredients, except for pasta and arugula. Stir until mixed and cook for 10 minutes until thickened.
3. When done, mash with the fork, top with arugula and serve with pasta. Serve straight away.

Nutrition:
- Calories: 236
- Fat: 1.6 g

- Carbohydrates: 46 g
- Protein: 12 g

Quinoa and Chickpeas Salad

Preparation Time: 10 minutes
Cooking Time: 0 minutes
Servings: 4
Ingredients:

- ¾ cup chopped broccoli
- ½ cup quinoa, cooked
- 15 ounces cooked chickpeas
- ½ teaspoon minced garlic
- ⅓ teaspoon ground black pepper
- ⅔ teaspoon salt
- 1 teaspoon dried tarragon
- 2 teaspoons mustard
- 1 tablespoon lemon juice
- 3 tablespoons olive oil

Directions:

1. Take a large bowl and put all the ingredients in it. Stir until well combined.
2. Serve straight away.

Nutrition:

- Calories: 264
- Fat: 12.3 g
- Carbohydrates: 32 g
- Protein: 7.1 g

Garlic and White Bean Soup

Preparation Time: 15 minutes
Cooking Time: 10 minutes
Servings: 4
Ingredients:

- 45 ounces cooked cannellini beans
- ¼ teaspoon dried thyme
- 2 teaspoons minced garlic
- ⅛ teaspoon crushed red pepper
- ½ teaspoon dried rosemary
- ⅛ teaspoon ground black pepper
- 2 tablespoons olive oil
- 4 cups vegetable broth

Directions:

1. Place one-third of white beans in a food processor. Then pour in 2 cups broth and pulse for 2 minutes until smooth.
2. Place a pot over medium heat. Add oil, and when hot, incorporate garlic and cook for 1 minute until fragrant.
3. Add pureed beans into the pan along with remaining beans. Sprinkle with spices and herbs and pour in the broth. Stir until combined and

bring the mixture to boil over medium-high heat.

4. Switch heat to medium-low level and simmer the beans for 15 minutes. Then mash them with a fork. Taste the soup to adjust seasoning and then serve.

Nutrition:

- Calories: 222
- Fat: 7 g
- Carbohydrates: 13 g
- Protein: 11.2 g

Coconut Curry Lentils

Preparation Time: 10 minutes
Cooking Time: 40 minutes
Servings: 4
Ingredients:

- 1 cup brown lentils
- 1 small white onion, peeled, chopped
- 1 teaspoon minced garlic
- 1 teaspoon grated ginger
- 3 cups baby spinach
- 1 tablespoon curry powder
- 2 tablespoons olive oil
- 13 ounces coconut milk, unsweetened
- 2 cups vegetable broth

For Serving:

- 4 cups cooked rice
- ¼ cup chopped cilantro

Directions:

1. Put oil in your large pot over medium heat, and when hot, add ginger and garlic. Cook for 1 minute until fragrant.
2. Add onion and cook for 5 minutes. Stir in curry powder. Cook for 1 minute until toasted; add lentils and pour in broth.
3. Switch heat to medium-high level and bring the mixture to a boil. Then switch heat to the low level and simmer for 20 minutes until tender and all the liquid is absorbed.
4. Pour in milk and stir until combined. Turn heat to medium level and simmer for 10 minutes until thickened.
5. Remove the pot and stir in spinach. Let it stand for 5 minutes until its leaves wilts, and then top with cilantro. Serve lentils with rice.

Nutrition:

- Calories: 184
- Fat: 3.7 g
- Carbohydrates: 30 g
- Protein: 11.3 g

Chard Wraps with Millet

Preparation Time: 25 minutes
Cooking Time: 0 minutes
Servings: 4
Ingredients:

- 1 carrot, cut into ribbons
- ½ cup millet, cooked
- ½ a large cucumber, cut into ribbons
- ½ cup chickpeas, cooked
- 1 cup sliced cabbage
- ⅓ cup hummus
- Mint leaves as needed for topping
- Hemp seeds as needed for topping
- 1 bunch Swiss rainbow chard

Directions:

1. Spread hummus on one side of chard and place some of the millet, vegetables, and chickpeas on it. Sprinkle with some mint leaves then hemp seeds and wrap it like a burrito.
2. Serve straight away.

Nutrition:

- Calories: 152 Fat: 4.5 g
- Carbohydrates: 25 g Protein: 3.5 g

Stuffed Peppers with Kidney Beans

Preparation Time: 5 minutes
Cooking Time: 35 minutes
Servings: 4
Ingredients:

- 3-½ ounces cooked kidney beans
- 1 big tomato, diced
- 3-½ ounces sweet corn, canned
- 2 medium bell peppers, deseeded, halved
- ½ medium red onion, peeled, diced
- 1 teaspoon garlic powder
- ⅓ teaspoon ground black pepper
- ⅔ teaspoon salt
- ½ teaspoon dried basil
- 3 teaspoons parsley
- ½ teaspoon dried thyme
- 3 tablespoons cashew
- 1 teaspoon olive oil

Directions:

1. Switch on the oven, then set it to 400°Fahrenheit and let it preheat. Take a large skillet pan and place it over medium heat. Add oil, and when hot, incorporate onion and cook for 2 minutes until translucent.
2. Add beans, tomatoes, and corn. Stir in garlic and cashews and cook for 5 minutes.

3. Stir in salt, black pepper, parsley, basil, and thyme. Remove the pan from heat and evenly divide the mixture between bell peppers. Bake the peppers for 25 minutes until tender; then top with parsley and serve.

Nutrition:

- Calories: 139 Fat: 1.6 g
- Carbohydrates: 18 g Protein: 5.1 g

Emmenthal Soup

Preparation Time: 15 minutes
Cooking Time: 0 minutes
Servings: 2
Ingredients:

- Picnh of Cayenne
- Pinch of Nutmeg
- 1 tablespoon pumpkin seeds
- 2 tablespoons chopped chives
- 3 tablespoons cubed emmenthal cheese
- 2 cups vegetable broth
- 1 cubed potato
- 2 cups cauliflower pieces

Directions:

1. Place the potato and cauliflower into a saucepan with the vegetable broth just until tender. Place into a blender and puree.
2. Add in spices and adjust to taste. Ladle into bowls, add in chives and cheese and stir well. Garnish with pumpkin seeds. Enjoy.

Nutrition:

- Calories: 380 Carbohydrates: 0 g
- Fat: 28 g Protein: 27 g

Pesto Quinoa with White Beans

Preparation Time: 5 minutes
Cooking Time: 15 minutes
Servings: 4
Ingredients:

- 12 ounces cooked white bean
- 3-½ cups quinoa, cooked
- 1 medium zucchini, sliced
- ¾ cup sun-dried tomato
- ¼ cup pine nuts
- 1 tablespoon olive oil

For the Pesto:

- ⅓ cup walnuts
- 2 cups arugula
- 1 teaspoon minced garlic
- 2 cups basil
- ¾ teaspoon salt
- ¼ teaspoon ground black pepper

- 1 tablespoon lemon juice
- $\frac{1}{3}$ cup olive oil
- 2 tablespoons water

Directions:
1. Prepare the pesto. Place all of its ingredients in a food processor and pulse for 2 minutes until smooth, scraping the sides of the container frequently, and set aside until required.
2. Take a large skillet pan and place it over medium heat. Add oil, and when hot, add zucchini and cook for 4 minutes until tender-crisp.
3. Season zucchini with salt and black pepper. Cook for 2 minutes until lightly brown. Add tomatoes and white beans and continue cooking for 4 minutes until white beans begin to crisp.
4. Stir in pine nuts and cook for 2 minutes until toasted. Remove the pan from heat and transfer the zucchini mixture into a medium bowl.
5. Add quinoa and pesto and stir until well combined; then distribute among four bowls and serve.

Nutrition:
- Calories: 352
- Fat: 27.3 g
- Carbohydrates: 33.7 g
- Protein: 9.7 g

Mushroom Leek Soup

Preparation Time: 15 minutes
Cooking Time: 20 minutes
Servings: 4
Ingredients:
- 1-½ tablespoons sherry vinegar
- ½ cup almond milk
- ¾ cup coconut cream
- 3 cups vegetable broth
- 1 tablespoon chopped dill
- Pepper to taste
- Salt, to taste
- 5 tablespoons almond flour
- 7 cups cleaned, sliced mushrooms
- 3 cloves minced garlic
- 2-¾ cups chopped leeks
- 3 tablespoons vegetable oil

Directions:
1. Place a Dutch oven on medium and warm the oil. Add in the leeks together with garlic bulb; then prepare till soft. Put in the mushrooms, stir and cook for an additional 10 minutes.
2. Add salt, dill, pepper, and flour. Stir well until combined. Put in soup and make it to simmer. Lower the heat and add in the rest of the

ingredients. Stir well. Cook an additional 10 minutes. Serve warm with almond flour bread.

Nutrition:
- Calories: 117
- Carbohydrates: 19 g
- Fat: 2 g
- Protein: 3 g

Fresh Veggie Pizza

Preparation Time: 15 minutes
Cooking Time: 14 minutes
Servings: 4
Ingredients:
Crust:
- ½ teaspoon garlic bulb flavored powder
- ½ teaspoon seawater salt
- 3 tablespoons coconut oil
- 1-¼ cups almond flour

Tahini-Bee Spread:
- A pinch pepper
- A pinch sea salt
- 2 garlic cloves
- 1 tablespoon lemon juice
- 1 tablespoon avocado oil
- 1 tablespoon Middle Eastern paste
- 2 peeled and cubed beets

Directions:
1. Start by placing your oven at 375°Fahrenheit. Place some parchment on a sheet tray. Stir together the salt, garlic powder, coconut oil, and almond flour.
2. Place this on the sheet tray and squeeze it into the shape of a ball. Place another piece of parchment on top and roll out the dough into a 7x7 square. Bake for 14 minutes, or until it starts to brown.
3. As the crust bakes, add the pepper, salt, garlic, lemon juice, avocado oil, tahini, and beets to a food processor. Mix until it becomes creamy.
4. To make your pizza, spread the crust with beet sauces and then top with your favorite alkaline-friendly veggies. Slice into four and enjoy.

Nutrition:
- Calories: 368 Carbohydrates: 46 g
- Fat: 13 g Protein: 16 g

Roasted Cauliflower Wraps

Preparation Time: 15 minutes
Cooking Time: 30-35 minutes
Servings: 2
Ingredients:
Cauliflower:
- ¼ teaspoon pepper

- ¼ teaspoon sea salt
- ½ teaspoon garlic powder
- ¼ cup nutritional yeast
- ¼ cup almond flour
- 1 tablespoon avocado oil
- 2 cups bite-size cauliflower florets

Sauce:
- Sea salt to taste
- 2 tablespoons apple cider vinegar
- 2 garlic cloves
- 1 Habanero pepper
- 1 cup cubed mango

Assembling:
- 2 leaves collard greens
- 1 cup mixed salad greens

Directions:
1. Start by placing your oven at 350°Fahrenheit and put a few papers on a cooking film. For your cauliflower, toss the cauliflower in the avocado oil and make sure they are evenly coated.
2. Into a container, combine along with all the pepper, salt, garlic powder, healthy fungus, together with the almond flour.
3. Sprinkle the breading over the cauliflower and toss everything together making sure the cauliflower is well-coated. Spread across the cooking film.
4. Cook it on about 30 up to 35 minutes, either that or till the cauliflower is soft.
5. As the cauliflower bakes, add the salt, vinegar, garlic, habanero, and mango to your blender and mix until well-combined.
6. Make sure you use some gloves or wash your hands really well when it comes to handling the habanero.
7. To assemble, divide the mixed salad greens between the collard leaves. Top with the cauliflower, and drizzle on the sauce. Wrap everything up like a burrito and enjoy.

Nutrition:
- Calories: 270
- Carbohydrates: 14 g
- Fat: 22 g
- Protein: 6 g

Pineapple, Papaya, and Mango Delight

Preparation Time: 15 minutes
Cooking Time: 0 minutes

Servings: 5
Ingredients:
- 1 pound fresh pineapple, peeled and cut into chunks
- 1 mango, peeled, pitted and cubed
- 2 papayas, peeled, seeded and cubed
- 3 tablespoons fresh lime juice
- ¼ cup fresh mint leaves, chopped

Directions:
1. Take a large bowl and add the listed ingredients. Toss well to coat. Put it in the fridge and let it chill. Serve and enjoy!

Nutrition:
- Calories: 292
- Fat: 11 g
- Carbohydrates: 42 g
- Protein: 8 g

BBQ Zucchini

Preparation Time: 15 minutes
Cooking Time: 60 minutes
Servings: 1
Ingredients:
- Olive oil as needed
- 3 zucchinis
- ½ teaspoon black pepper
- ½ teaspoon mustard
- ½ teaspoon cumin
- 1 teaspoon paprika
- 1 teaspoon garlic powder
- 1 tablespoon sea salt
- 1-2 stevia
- 1 tablespoon chili powder

Directions:
1. Preheat your oven to 300°Fahrenheit. Take a small bowl and add cayenne, black pepper, salt, garlic, mustard, paprika, chili powder, and stevia. Mix well.
2. Slice zucchini into ⅛-inch slices and mist them with olive oil. Sprinkle spice blend over zucchini and bake for 40 minutes.
3. Remove and flip, mist with more olive oil and leftover spice. Bake for 20 minutes more. Serve!

Nutrition:
- Calories: 163
- Fat: 14 g
- Carbohydrates: 3 g
- Protein: 8 g

Grilled Eggplant Steaks

Preparation Time: 15 minutes

Cooking Time: 10 minutes
Servings: 4
Ingredients:

- 4 Roma tomatoes, diced
- 8 ounces cashew cream
- 2 eggplants
- 1 tablespoon olive oil
- 1 cup parsley, chopped
- 1 cucumber, diced
- Salt and pepper to taste

Directions:

1. Slice eggplants into three thick steaks, drizzle with oil, and season with salt and pepper. Grill in a pan for 4 minutes per side. Top with remaining ingredients. Serve and enjoy!

Nutrition:

- Calories: 86
- Fat: 7 g
- Carbohydrates: 12 g
- Protein: 8 g

Garlic Zucchini and Cauliflower

Preparation Time: 10 minutes
Cooking Time: 20 minutes
Servings: 4
Ingredients:

- 4 zucchinis, cut into medium fries
- 1 cup cauliflower florets
- 1 tablespoon capers, drained
- ½ lemon juice
- A pinch salt and black pepper
- ½ teaspoon chili powder
- 1 tablespoon olive oil
- ¼ teaspoon garlic powder

Directions:

1. Spread the zucchini fries on a lined baking sheet. Add the rest of the ingredients. Toss,

introduce in the oven and bake at 400°Fahrenheit for 20 minutes. Divide between plates and serve.

Nutrition:

- Calories: 185
- Fat: 3 g
- Carbohydrates: 6.5 g
- Protein: 8 g

Garlic Beans

Preparation Time: 10 minutes
Cooking Time: 10 minutes
Servings: 4
Ingredients:

- 1 lemon juice
- 1 lemon zest, grated
- 2 tablespoons avocado oil
- 4 garlic cloves, minced
- ½ teaspoon turmeric powder
- 1 teaspoon garam masala
- 1 red onion, sliced
- 1 yellow bell pepper, sliced
- 10 ounces green beans, halved
- A pinch black pepper

Directions:

1. Warm up a pan with the oil over medium-high heat. Add the garlic and onion and cook for 2 minutes.
2. Add green beans and the other ingredients, toss, cook for 8 minutes, divide between plates and serve.

Nutrition:

- Calories: 180 Fat: 10 g
- Carbohydrates: 13 g
- Protein: 8 g

Chapter 6:   Vegetables & Side Dishes

Easy & Crispy Brussels Sprouts

Preparation Time: 10 minutes
Cooking Time: 15 minutes
Servings: 4
Ingredients:

- 2 cups Brussels sprouts
- 2 tablespoons everything bagel seasoning
- ¼ cup almonds, crushed
- ¼ cup parmesan cheese, grated
- 2 tablespoons olive oil
- 2 cups water
- Salt to taste

Directions:

1. Add Brussels sprouts into the saucepan with 2 cups of water. Cover and cook for 8-10 minutes.
2. Drain well and allow to cool completely. Slice each Brussels sprouts in half.
3. Add Brussels sprouts and remaining ingredients into the mixing bowl and toss to coat.
4. Add Brussels sprout mixture into the Air Fryer basket and cook at 375°Fahrenheit for 12-15 minutes.
5. Serve and enjoy.

Nutrition:

- Calories: 144
- Fat: 11.5 g
- Carbohydrates: 7.6 g
- Sugar 1.4 g
- Protein: 5.1 g
- Cholesterol 4 mg

Garlic Green Beans

Preparation Time: 10 minutes
Cooking Time: 8 minutes
Servings: 4
Ingredients:

- 1 pound fresh green beans, trimmed
- 1 teaspoon garlic powder
- 1 tablespoon olive oil
- Pepper to taste
- Salt to taste

Directions:

1. Drizzle green beans with oil and season with garlic powder, pepper, and salt.

2. Place green beans into the Air Fryer basket and cook at 370°Fahrenheit for 8 minutes. Toss halfway through.
3. Serve and enjoy.

Nutrition:

- Calories: 68
- Fat: 3.7 g
- Carbohydrates: 8.6 g
- Sugar 1.8 g
- Protein: 2.2 g
- Cholesterol 0 mg

Simple Vegan Broccoli

Preparation Time: 10 minutes
Cooking Time: 5 minutes
Servings: 2
Ingredients:

- 4 cups broccoli florets
- 1 tablespoon nutritional yeast
- 2 tablespoons olive oil
- Pepper to taste
- Salt to taste

Directions:

1. In a medium bowl, mix together broccoli, nutritional yeast, oil, pepper, and salt.
2. Add broccoli florets into the Air Fryer basket and cook at 370°Fahrenheit for 5 minutes.
3. Serve and enjoy.

Nutrition:

- Calories: 158 Fat: 14.3 g
- Carbohydrates: 6.3 g Sugar 1 g
- Protein: 4.3 g Cholesterol 0 mg

Asparagus with Almonds

Preparation Time: 10 minutes
Cooking Time: 5 minutes
Servings: 4
Ingredients:

- 12 asparagus spears
- ⅓ cup sliced almonds
- 2 tablespoons olive oil
- 2 tablespoons balsamic vinegar
- Pepper to taste
- Salt to taste

Directions:

1. Drizzle asparagus spears with oil and vinegar.

2. Arrange asparagus spears into the Air Fryer basket and season with pepper and salt.
3. Sprinkle sliced almond over asparagus spears.
4. Cook asparagus at 350°Fahrenheit for 5 minutes. Shake basket halfway through.
5. Serve and enjoy.

Nutrition:
- Calories: 122
- Fat: 11.1 g
- Carbohydrates: 4.6 g
- Sugar 1.7 g
- Protein: 3.3 g
- Cholesterol 0 mg

Easy Roasted Carrots

Preparation Time: 10 minutes
Cooking Time: 18 minutes
Servings: 4
Ingredients:
- 16 ounces carrots, peeled and cut into 2-inch chunks
- 1 teaspoon olive oil
- Pepper to taste
- Salt to taste

Directions:
1. Preheat the cosori Air Fryer to 360°Fahrenheit.
2. Toss carrots with oil and season with pepper and salt.
3. Add carrots into the Air Fryer basket and cook for 15-18 minutes. Shake basket 3-4 times.
4. Serve and enjoy.

Nutrition:
- Calories: 57
- Fat: 1.2 g
- Carbohydrates: 11.2 g
- Sugar 5.6 g
- Protein: 0.9 g
- Cholesterol 0 mg

Asian Broccoli

Preparation Time: 10 minutes
Cooking Time: 20 minutes
Servings: 4
Ingredients:
- 1 pound broccoli florets
- 1 teaspoon rice vinegar
- 2 teaspoons sriracha
- 2 tablespoons soy sauce
- 1 tablespoon garlic, minced
- 1-½ tablespoons sesame oil
- Salt to taste

Directions:

1. Toss broccoli florets with garlic, sesame oil, and salt.
2. Add broccoli florets into the Air Fryer basket and cook at 400°Fahrenheit for 15-20 minutes. Shake basket halfway through.
3. In a mixing bowl, mix together rice vinegar, sriracha, and soy sauce. Add broccoli and toss well.
4. Serve and enjoy.

Nutrition:
- Calories: 94
- Fat: 5.5 g
- Carbohydrates: 9.3 g
- Sugar 2.1 g
- Protein: 3.8 g
- Cholesterol 0 mg

Healthy Squash & Zucchini

Preparation Time: 10 minutes
Cooking Time: 25 minutes
Servings: 4
Ingredients:
- 1 pound zucchini, cut into ½-inch half-moons
- 1 pound yellow squash, cut into ½-inch half-moons
- 1 tablespoon olive oil
- Pepper to taste
- Salt to taste

Directions:
1. In a mixing bowl, add zucchini, squash, oil, pepper, and salt and toss well.
2. Add zucchini and squash mixture into the Air Fryer basket and cook at 400°Fahrenheit for 20 minutes. Shake basket halfway through.
3. Shake basket well and cook for 5 minutes more.
4. Serve and enjoy.

Nutrition:
- Calories: 66
- Fat: 3.9 g
- Carbohydrates: 7.6 g
- Sugar 3.9 g
- Protein: 2.7 g
- Cholesterol 0 mg

Crunchy Fried Cabbage

Preparation Time: 10 minutes
Cooking Time: 10 minutes
Servings: 2
Ingredients:
- ½ cabbage head, sliced into 2-inch slices
- 1 tablespoon olive oil
- Pepper to taste
- Salt to taste

Directions:
1. Drizzle cabbage with olive oil and season with pepper and salt.
2. Add cabbage slices into the Air Fryer basket and cook at 375°Fahrenheit for 5 minutes.
3. Toss cabbage well and cook for 5 minutes more.
4. Serve and enjoy.

Nutrition:
- Calories: 105
- Fat: 7.2 g
- Carbohydrates: 10.4 g
- Sugar 5.7 g
- Protein: 2.3 g
- Cholesterol 0 mg

Quick Vegetable Kebabs

Preparation Time: 10 minutes
Cooking Time: 10 minutes
Servings: 4
Ingredients:
- 2 bell peppers, cut into 1-inch pieces
- ½ onion, cut into 1-inch pieces
- 1 zucchini, cut into 1-inch pieces
- 1 eggplant, cut into 1-inch pieces
- Pepper to taste
- Salt to taste

Directions:
1. Thread vegetables onto the skewers and spray them with cooking spray. Season with pepper and salt.
2. Preheat the Cosori Air Fryer to 390 Fahrenheit.
3. Place skewers into the Air Fryer basket and cooks for 10 minutes. Turn halfway through.
4. Serve and enjoy.

Nutrition:
- Calories: 48
- Fat: 0.3 g
- Carbohydrates: 11.2 g
- Sugar 5.9 g
- Protein: 2.1 g
- Cholesterol 0 mg

Easy Soy Garlic Mushrooms

Preparation Time: 10 minutes
Cooking Time: 12 minutes
Servings: 2
Ingredients:
- 8 ounces mushrooms, cleaned
- 1 tablespoon fresh parsley, chopped
- 1 teaspoon soy sauce

- ½ teaspoon garlic powder
- 1 tablespoon olive oil
- Pepper to taste
- Salt to taste

Directions:
1. Toss mushrooms with soy sauce, garlic powder, oil, pepper, and salt.
2. Add mushrooms into the Air Fryer basket and cook at 380°Fahrenheit for 10-12 minutes.
3. Garnish with parsley and serve.

Nutrition:
- Calories: 89
- Fat: 7.4 g
- Carbohydrates: 4.6 g
- Sugar 2.2 g
- Protein: 3.9 g
- Cholesterol 0 mg

Spicy Edamame

Preparation Time: 10 minutes
Cooking Time: 18 minutes
Servings: 4
Ingredients:
- 16 ounces frozen edamame in shell, defrosted
- 1 lemon juice
- 1 lemon zest
- 1 tablespoon garlic, sliced
- 2 teaspoons olive oil
- ½ teaspoon chili powder
- ½ teaspoon paprika
- Salt to taste

Directions:
1. Toss edamame with lemon zest, garlic, oil, chili powder, paprika, and salt.
2. Add edamame into the Air Fryer basket and cook at 400°Fahrenheit for 18 minutes. Shake basket twice.
3. Drizzle lemon juice over edamame and serve.

Nutrition:
- Calories: 172
- Fat: 8.5 g
- Carbohydrates: 12.2 g
- Sugar 2.7 g
- Protein: 12.3 g
- Cholesterol 0 mg

Balsamic Mushrooms

Preparation Time: 10 minutes
Cooking Time: 8 minutes
Servings: 3
Ingredients:

- 8 ounces mushrooms
- 1 teaspoon fresh parsley, chopped
- 2 teaspoons balsamic vinegar
- ½ teaspoon granulated garlic
- 1 teaspoon olive oil
- Pepper to taste
- Salt to taste

Directions:

1. Toss mushrooms with garlic, oil, pepper, and salt.
2. Add mushrooms into the Air Fryer basket and cook at 375°Fahrenheit for 8 minutes. Toss halfway through.
3. Toss mushrooms with parsley and balsamic vinegar.
4. Serve and enjoy.

Nutrition:

- Calories: 32 Fat: 1.8 g
- Carbohydrates: 2.9 g Sugar 1.4 g
- Protein: 2.5 g
- Cholesterol 0 mg

Mediterranean Vegetables

Preparation Time: 10 minutes
Cooking Time: 15 minutes
Servings: 2
Ingredients:

- 6 cherry tomatoes, cut in half
- 1 eggplant, diced
- 1 zucchini, diced
- 1 green bell pepper, diced
- 1 teaspoon thyme
- 1 teaspoon oregano
- Pepper to taste
- Salt to taste

Directions:

1. In a bowl, toss eggplant, zucchini, bell pepper, thyme, oregano, pepper, and salt.
2. Add vegetable mixture into the Air Fryer basket and cook at 360°Fahrenheit for 12 minutes.
3. Add cherry tomatoes and shake basket well and cook for 3 minutes more.
4. Serve and enjoy.

Nutrition:

- Calories: 61
- Fat: 0.3 g
- Carbohydrates: 13.8 g
- Sugar 7.6 g
- Protein: 2.8 g
- Cholesterol 0 mg

Simple Roasted Okra

Preparation Time: 10 minutes
Cooking Time: 12 minutes
Servings: 1
Ingredients:

- ½ pound okra, trimmed and sliced
- 1 teaspoon olive oil
- Pepper to taste
- Salt to taste

Directions:

1. Preheat the Cosori Air Fryer to 350°Fahrenheit.
2. Mix together okra, oil, pepper, and salt.
3. Add okra into the Air Fryer basket and cook for 10 minutes. Toss halfway through.
4. Toss well and cook for 2 minutes more.
5. Serve and enjoy.

Nutrition:

- Calories: 176
- Fat: 17.3 g
- Carbohydrates: 6.2 g
- Sugar 3.2 g
- Protein: 2.5 g
- Cholesterol 0 mg

Hydrated Potato Wedges

Preparation Time: 5 minutes
Cooking Time: 30 minutes
Servings: 5
Ingredients:

- 2 medium Russet potatoes, diced into wedges
- 1-½ tablespoons olive oil
- ½ teaspoon chili powder
- ½ teaspoon parsley
- ½ teaspoon paprika
- ⅛ teaspoon black pepper
- ½ teaspoon sea salt

Directions:

1. In a large bowl, mix potato wedges, olive oil, chili, parsley, paprika, salt, and pepper until the potatoes are well coated.
2. Transfer half of the potatoes to a fryer basket and hydrate for 20 minutes.
3. Repeat with the remaining wedges. Serve hot with chilled orange juice.

Nutrition:

- Calories129
- Carbohydrates: 10 g
- Fat: 5.3 g
- Protein: 2.3 g

Hydrated Kale Chips

Preparation Time: 5 minutes

Cooking Time: 5 minutes
Servings: 2
Ingredients:
- 4 cups loosely packed kale, stemmed
- 2 teaspoons ranch seasoning
- 2 tablespoons olive oil
- 1 tablespoon nutritional yeast
- ¼ teaspoon salt

Directions:
1. In a bowl, toss together kale pieces, oil, nutritional yeast, ranch seasoning, and salt until well coated.
2. Transfer to a fryer basket and hydrate for 15 minutes, shaking halfway through cooking.
3. Serve right away!

Nutrition:
- Calories: 103
- Carbohydrates: 8.2 g
- Fat: 7.1 g
- Protein: 3.2 g

Greek Vegetables

Preparation Time: 10 minutes
Cooking Time: 20 minutes
Servings: 4
Ingredients:
- 1 carrot, sliced
- 1 parsnip, sliced
- 1 green bell pepper, chopped
- 1 courgette, chopped
- ¼ cup cherry tomatoes, cut in half
- 6 tablespoons olive oil
- 2 teaspoons garlic puree
- 1 teaspoon mustard
- 1 teaspoon mixed herbs
- Pepper to taste
- Salt to taste

Directions:
1. Add cherry tomatoes, carrot, parsnip, bell pepper, and courgette into the Air Fryer basket.
2. Drizzle olive oil over vegetables and cook at 350°Fahrenheitfor 15 minutes.
3. In a mixing bowl, mix together the remaining ingredients. Add vegetables into the mixing bowl and toss well.
4. Return vegetables to the Air Fryer basket and cook at 400°Fahrenheitfor 5 minutes more.
5. Serve and enjoy.

Nutrition:
- Calories: 66 Fat: 1.5 g
- Carbohydrates: 12.7 g

- Sugar 5.3 g
- Protein: 1.8 g
- Cholesterol 1 mg

Lemon Garlic Cauliflower

Preparation Time: 10 minutes
Cooking Time: 10 minutes
Servings: 2
Ingredients:
- 3 cups cauliflower
- 1 tablespoon fresh parsley, chopped
- ½ teaspoon lemon juice
- 1 tablespoon pine nuts
- ½ teaspoon dried oregano
- 1-½ teaspoons olive oil
- Pepper to taste
- Salt to taste

Directions:
1. Add cauliflower, oregano, oil, pepper, and salt into the mixing bowl and toss well.
2. Add cauliflower into the Air Fryer basket and cook at 375°Fahrenheit for 10 minutes.
3. Transfer cauliflower into the serving bowl. Add pine nuts, parsley, and lemon juice, and toss well.
4. Serve and enjoy.

Nutrition:
- Calories: 99 Fat: 6.7 g
- Carbohydrates: 8.9 g
- Sugar 3.8 g
- Protein: 3.7 g
- Cholesterol 0 mg

Balsamic Brussels Sprouts

Preparation Time: 10 minutes
Cooking Time: 20 minutes
Servings: 4
Ingredients:
- 1 pound Brussels sprouts, remove ends and cut in half
- 1 tablespoon balsamic vinegar
- 2 tablespoons olive oil
- Pepper to taste
- Salt to taste

Directions:
1. Add Brussels sprouts, vinegar, oil, pepper, and salt into the mixing bowl and toss well.
2. Add Brussels sprouts into the Air Fryer basket and cook at 360°Fahrenheit for 15-20 minutes. Toss halfway through.
3. Serve and enjoy.

Nutrition:
- Calories: 110
- Fat: 7.4 g
- Carbohydrates: 10.4 g
- Sugar 2.5 g
- Protein: 3.9 g
- Cholesterol 0 mg

Flavorful Butternut Squash

Preparation Time: 10 minutes
Cooking Time: 15 minutes
Servings: 4
Ingredients:
- 4 cups butternut squash, cut into 1-inch pieces
- 1 teaspoon Chinese five-spice powder
- 1 tablespoon Truvia
- 2 tablespoon olive oil

Directions:
1. Add butternut squash and remaining ingredients into the mixing bowl and mix well.
2. Add butternut squash into the Air Fryer basket and cook at 400°Fahrenheitfor 15 minutes. Shake basket halfway through.
3. Serve and enjoy.

Nutrition:
- Calories: 83
- Fat: 7.1 g
- Carbohydrates: 6.7 g
- Sugar 2.2 g
- Protein: 0.6 g
- Cholesterol 0 mg

Crispy Green Beans

Preparation Time: 10 minutes
Cooking Time: 10 minutes
Servings: 4
Ingredients:
- 2 cups green beans, ends trimmed
- 2 tablespoons parmesan cheese, shredded
- 1 tablespoon fresh lemon juice
- 1 teaspoon Italian seasoning
- 2 teaspoons olive oil
- ¼ teaspoon salt

Directions:
1. Preheat the cosori Air Fryer to 400°Fahrenheit.
2. Brush green beans with olive oil and season with Italian seasoning and salt.
3. Place green beans into the Air Fryer basket and cook for 8-10 minutes. Shake basket 2-3 times.
4. Transfer green beans to a serving plate.
5. Pour lemon juice over beans and sprinkle shredded cheese on top of beans.

6. Serve and enjoy.

Nutrition:
- Calories: 64
- Fat: 4.3 g
- Carbohydrates: 4.4 g
- Sugar 1 g
- Protein: 3.3 g
- Cholesterol 6 mg

Roasted Zucchini

Preparation Time: 10 minutes
Cooking Time: 10 minutes
Servings: 4
Ingredients:
- 2 medium zucchini, cut into 1-inch slices
- 1 teaspoon lemon zest
- 1 tablespoon olive oil
- Pepper to taste
- Salt to taste

Directions:
1. Toss zucchini with lemon zest, oil, pepper, and salt.
2. Arrange zucchini slices into the Air Fryer basket and cook at 350°Fahrenheitfor 10 minutes. Turn halfway through.
3. Serve and enjoy.

Nutrition:
- Calories: 46 Fat: 3.7 g
- Carbohydrates: 3.4 g Sugar 1.7 g
- Protein: 1.2 g Cholesterol 0 mg

Crispy & Spicy Eggplant

Preparation Time: 10 minutes
Cooking Time: 20 minutes
Servings: 4
Ingredients:
- 1 eggplant, cut into 1-inch pieces
- ½ teaspoon Italian seasoning
- 1 teaspoon paprika
- ½ teaspoon red pepper
- 1 teaspoon garlic powder
- 2 tablespoons olive oil

Directions:
1. Add eggplant and remaining ingredients into the bowl and toss well.
2. Spray Air Fryer basket with cooking spray.
3. Add eggplant into the Air Fryer basket and cook at 375°Fahrenheit for 20 minutes. Shake basket halfway through.
4. Serve and enjoy.

Nutrition:

- Calories: 99
- Fat: 7.5 g
- Carbohydrates: 8.7 g
- Sugar 4.5 g
- Protein: 1.5 g
- Cholesterol 0 mg

Spiced Green Beans

Preparation Time: 10 minutes
Cooking Time: 10 minutes
Servings: 2
Ingredients:
- 2 cups green beans
- $\frac{1}{8}$ teaspoon ground allspice
- ¼ teaspoon ground cinnamon
- ½ teaspoon dried oregano
- 2 tablespoon olive oil
- ¼ teaspoon ground coriander
- ¼ teaspoon ground cumin
- $\frac{1}{8}$ teaspoon cayenne pepper
- ½ teaspoon salt

Directions:
1. Add all ingredients into the medium bowl and toss well.
2. Oil Air Fryer basket with cooking spray.
3. Add green beans into the Air Fryer basket and cook at 370°Fahrenheit for 10 minutes. Shake basket halfway through.
4. Serve and enjoy.

Nutrition:
- Calories: 158
- Fat: 14.3 g
- Carbohydrates: 8.6 g
- Sugar 1.6 g
- Protein: 2.1 g
- Cholesterol 0 mg

Air Fryer Basil Tomatoes

Preparation Time: 10 minutes
Cooking Time: 25 minutes
Servings: 4
Ingredients:
- 4 large tomatoes, halved
- 1 garlic clove, minced
- 1 tablespoon vinegar
- 1 tablespoon olive oil
- 2 tablespoons parmesan cheese, grated
- ½ teaspoon fresh parsley, chopped
- 1 teaspoon fresh basil, minced
- Pepper to taste

- Salt to taste

Directions:
1. Preheat the Cosori Air Fryer to 320°Fahrenheit.
2. In a bowl, mix together oil, basil, garlic, vinegar, pepper, and salt. Add tomatoes and stir to coat.
3. Place tomato halves into the Air Fryer basket and cook for 20 minutes.
4. Sprinkle parmesan cheese over tomatoes and cook for 5 minutes more.
5. Serve and enjoy.

Nutrition:
- Calories: 87
- Fat: 5.4 g
- Carbohydrates: 7.7 g
- Sugar 4.8 g
- Protein: 3.9 g
- Cholesterol 5 mg

Air Fryer Ratatouille

Preparation Time: 10 minutes
Cooking Time: 15 minutes
Servings: 6
Ingredients:
- 1 eggplant, diced
- 1 onion, diced
- 3 tomatoes, diced
- 1 red bell pepper, diced
- 1 green bell pepper, diced
- 1 tablespoon vinegar
- 2 tablespoons olive oil
- 2 tablespoons herb Provence
- 2 garlic cloves, chopped
- Pepper to taste
- Salt to taste

Directions:
1. Preheat the Cosori Air Fryer to 400°Fahrenheit.
2. Add all ingredients into the bowl and toss well and transfer into the Air Fryer safe dish.
3. Place dish into the Air Fryer basket and cook for 15 minutes. Stir halfway through.
4. Serve and enjoy.

Nutrition:
- Calories: 91
- Fat: 5 g
- Carbohydrates: 11.6 g
- Sugar 6.4 g
- Protein: 1.9 g
- Cholesterol 0 mg

Garlicky Cauliflower Florets

Preparation Time: 10 minutes
Cooking Time: 20 minutes
Servings: 4
Ingredients:

- 5 cups cauliflower florets
- ½ teaspoon cumin powder
- ½ teaspoon ground coriander
- 6 garlic cloves, chopped
- 4 tablespoons olive oil
- ½ teaspoon salt

Directions:

1. Add cauliflower florets and remaining ingredients into the large mixing bowl and toss well.
2. Add cauliflower florets into the Air Fryer basket and cook at 400°Fahrenheit for 20 minutes. Shake basket halfway through.
3. Serve and enjoy.

Nutrition:

- Calories: 159
- Fat: 14.2 g
- Carbohydrates: 8.2 g
- Sugar 3.1 g
- Protein: 2.8 g
- Cholesterol 0 mg

Parmesan Brussels Sprouts

Preparation Time: 10 minutes
Cooking Time: 12 minutes
Servings: 4
Ingredients:

- 1 pound Brussels sprouts, remove stems and halved
- ¼ cup parmesan cheese, grated
- 2 tablespoons olive oil
- Pepper to taste
- Salt to taste

Directions:

1. Preheat the cosori Air Fryer to 350°Fahrenheit.
2. In a mixing bowl, toss Brussels sprouts with oil, pepper, and salt.
3. Transfer Brussels sprouts into the Air Fryer basket and cooks for 12 minutes. Shake basket halfway through.
4. Sprinkle with parmesan cheese and serve.

Nutrition:

- Calories: 129 Fat: 8.7 g
- Carbohydrates: 10.6 g
- Sugar 2.5 g
- Protein: 5.9 g

- Cholesterol 4 mg

Flavorful Tomatoes

Preparation Time: 10 minutes
Cooking Time: 15 minutes
Servings: 4
Ingredients:

- 4 Roma tomatoes, sliced, remove seeds pithy portion
- 1 tablespoon olive oil
- ½ teaspoon dried thyme
- 2 garlic cloves, minced
- Pepper to taste
- Salt to taste

Directions:

1. Preheat the Cosori Air Fryer to 390°Fahrenheit.
2. Toss sliced tomatoes with oil, thyme, garlic, pepper, and salt.
3. Arrange sliced tomatoes into the Air Fryer basket and cook for 15 minutes.
4. Serve and enjoy.

Nutrition:

- Calories: 55
- Fat: 3.8 g
- Carbohydrates: 5.4 g
- Sugar 3.3 g
- Protein: 1.2 g
- Cholesterol 0 mg

Healthy Roasted Carrots

Preparation Time: 10 minutes
Cooking Time: 12 minutes
Servings: 4
Ingredients:

- 2 cups carrots, peeled and chopped
- 1 teaspoon cumin
- 1 tablespoon olive oil
- ¼ fresh coriander, chopped

Directions:

1. Toss carrots with cumin and oil and place them into the Air Fryer basket.
2. Cook at 390°Fahrenheit for 12 minutes.
3. Garnish with fresh coriander and serve.

Nutrition:

- Calories: 55
- Fat: 3.6 g
- Carbohydrates: 5.7 g
- Sugar 2.7 g
- Protein: 0.6 g
- Cholesterol 0 mg

Curried Cauliflower with Pine Nuts

Preparation Time: 10 minutes
Cooking Time: 10 minutes
Servings: 4
Ingredients:
- 1 small cauliflower head, cut into florets
- 2 tablespoons olive oil
- ¼ cup pine nuts, toasted
- 1 tablespoon curry powder
- ¼ teaspoon salt

Directions:
1. Preheat the Cosori Air Fryer to 350°Fahrenheit.
2. In a mixing bowl, toss cauliflower florets with oil, curry powder, and salt.
3. Add cauliflower florets into the Air Fryer basket and cook for 10 minutes. Shake basket halfway through.
4. Transfer cauliflower into the serving bowl. Add pine nuts and toss well.
5. Serve and enjoy.

Nutrition:
- Calories: 139
- Fat: 13.1 g
- Carbohydrates: 5.5 g
- Sugar 1.9 g
- Protein: 2.7 g
- Cholesterol 0 mg

Thyme Sage Butternut Squash

Preparation Time: 10 minutes
Cooking Time: 12 minutes
Servings: 4
Ingredients:
- 2 pounds butternut squash, cut into chunks
- 1 teaspoon fresh thyme, chopped
- 1 tablespoon fresh sage, chopped
- 1 tablespoon olive oil
- Pepper to taste
- Salt to taste

Directions:
1. Preheat the Cosori Air Fryer to 390°Fahrenheit.
2. In a mixing bowl, toss butternut squash with thyme, sage, oil, pepper, and salt.
3. Add butternut squash into the Air Fryer basket and cook for 10 minutes. Shake basket well and cook for 2 minutes more.
4. Serve and enjoy.

Nutrition:
- Calories: 50
- Fat: 3.8 g
- Carbohydrates: 4.2 g
- Sugar 2.5 g
- Protein: 1.4 g
- Cholesterol 0 mg

Guacamole

Preparation Time: 15 minutes
Cooking Time: 4 minutes
Servings: 4
Ingredients:
- 2 ripe avocados, halved and pitted
- 2 teaspoons vegetable oil
- 3 tablespoons fresh lime juice
- 1 garlic clove, crushed
- ¼ teaspoon ground chipotle chile
- Salt, as required
- ¼ cup red onion, chopped finely
- ¼ cup fresh cilantro, chopped finely

Directions:
1. Brush the cut sides of each avocado half with oil.
2. Place the water tray in the bottom of the Power XL Smokeless Electric Grill.
3. Place about 2 cups of lukewarm water into the water tray.
4. Place the drip pan over the water tray and then arrange the heating element.
5. Now, place the grilling pan overheating element.
6. Plugin the Power XL Smokeless Electric Grill and press the "Power" button to turn it on.
7. Then press the "Fan" button.
8. Set the temperature settings according to the manufacturer's directions.
9. Cover the grill with a lid and let it preheat.
10. After preheating, remove the lid and grease the grilling pan.
11. Place the avocado halves over the grilling pan, cut side down.
12. Cook, uncovered for about 2-4 minutes.
13. Transfer the avocados onto the cutting board and let them cool slightly.
14. Remove the peel and transfer the flesh into a bowl.
15. Add the lime juice, garlic, chipotle, and salt then with a fork, mash until almost smooth.
16. Stir in onion and cilantro and refrigerate, covered for about 1 hour before serving.

Nutrition:
- Calories: 230
- Fat: 21.9 g
- Saturated fat 4.6 g
- Cholesterol 0 mg

- Sodium 46 mg
- Carbohydrates: 9.7 g
- Fiber 6.9 g
- Sugar 0.8 g
- Protein: 2.1 g

Roasted Brussels Sprouts

Preparation Time: 30 minutes
Cooking Time: 20 minutes
Servings: 4
Ingredients:

- 1 pound Brussels sprouts, sliced in half
- 1 shallot, chopped
- 1 tablespoon olive oil
- Salt and pepper to taste
- 2 teaspoons balsamic vinegar
- ¼ cup pomegranate seeds
- ¼ cup goat cheese, crumbled

Directions:

1. Preheat your oven to 400°Fahrenheit.
2. Coat the Brussels sprouts with oil.
3. Sprinkle with salt and pepper.
4. Transfer to a baking pan.
5. Roast in the oven for 20 minutes.
6. Drizzle with vinegar.
7. Sprinkle with the seeds and cheese before serving.

Nutrition:

- Calories: 117 Fiber 4.8 g Protein: 5.8 g

Chapter 7:   Rice, Legumes & Grains

Veggie Sushi Bowl

Preparation Time: 15 minutes
Cooking Time: 10 minutes
Servings: 4
Ingredients:

- ½ cup Edamame beans, shelled and fresh
- ¾ cup brown rice, cooked
- ½ cup spinach, chopped
- ¼ cup bell pepper, sliced
- ¼ cup avocado, sliced
- ¼ cup cilantro, fresh and chopped
- 1 scallion, chopped
- ¼ nori sheet
- 1-2 tablespoons tamari
- 1 tablespoon sesame seeds

Directions:

1. Steam edamame beans as required. Take a bowl and add edamame, rice, avocado, spinach, cilantro, scallions, and bell pepper, and stir.
2. Cut nori into ribbons sprinkle the mixture on top. Drizzle it with tamari and sesame. Serve and enjoy!

Nutrition:

- Calories: 470 Fat: 20 g
- Carbohydrates: 50 g Protein: 22 g

Coconut Rice

Preparation Time: 10 minutes
Cooking Time: 25 minutes
Servings: 7
Ingredients:

- 2-½ cups white rice
- $1/8$ teaspoon salt
- 40 ounces coconut milk, unsweetened

Directions:

1. Take a large saucepan, place it over medium heat, add all the ingredients in it and stir until mixed.
2. Boil the mixture, then switch heat to medium-low level and simmer rice for 25 minutes until tender and all the liquid is absorbed. Serve straight away.

Nutrition:

- Calories: 535
- Fat: 33.2 g
- Carbohydrates: 57 g

- Protein: 8.1 g

Lentil, Rice and Vegetable Bake

Preparation Time: 10 minutes
Cooking Time: 40 minutes
Servings: 6
Ingredients:

- ½ cup white rice, cooked
- 1 cup red lentils, cooked
- $1/3$ cup chopped carrots
- 1 medium tomato, chopped
- 1 small onion, peeled, chopped
- $1/3$ cup chopped zucchini
- $1/3$ cup chopped celery
- 1-½ teaspoons minced garlic
- ½ teaspoon ground black pepper
- 1 teaspoon dried basil
- 1 teaspoon ground cumin
- 1 teaspoon dried oregano
- ½ teaspoon salt
- 1 teaspoon olive oil
- 8 ounces tomato sauce

Directions:

1. Take a skillet pan, place it over medium heat, add oil. When hot, add onion and garlic. Then cook for 5 minutes.
2. Add remaining vegetables. Season with salt, black pepper, and half of each cumin, oregano, and basil. Then cook for 5 minutes until vegetables are tender.
3. Take a casserole dish and place lentils and rice in it. Top with vegetables, spread with tomato sauce, and sprinkle with remaining cumin, oregano, and basil. Bake for 30 minutes until bubbly. Serve straight away.

Nutrition:

- Calories: 187 Fat: 1.5 g
- Carbohydrates: 35.1 g
- Protein: 9.7 g

Brown Rice Tabbouleh

Preparation Time: 20 minutes
Cooking Time: 0 minutes
Servings: 6
Ingredients:

- 3 cups brown rice, cooked
- ¾ cup cucumber, chopped

- ¾ cup tomato, chopped
- ¼ cup mint leaves, chopped
- ¼ cup green onions, sliced
- ¼ cup olive oil
- ¼ cup lemon juice
- Salt and pepper, to taste

Directions:

1. Combine all ingredients in a large bowl. Toss well and chill for 20 minutes.

Nutrition:

- Calories: 201
- Carbohydrates: 25 g
- Fat: 10 g
- Protein: 3 g

Black-Eyed Pea, Beet, and Carrot Stew

Preparation Time: 15 minutes
Cooking Time: 40 minutes
Servings: 2
Ingredients:

- ½ cup black-eyed peas, soaked in water overnight
- 3 cups water
- 1 large beet, peeled and cut into ½-inch pieces (about ¾ cup)
- 1 large carrot, peeled and cut into ½-inch pieces (about ¾ cup)
- ¼ teaspoon turmeric
- ¼ teaspoon toasted and ground cumin seeds
- ⅛ teaspoon asafetida
- ¼ cup finely chopped parsley
- ¼ teaspoon cayenne pepper
- ¼ teaspoon salt (optional)
- ½ teaspoon fresh lime juice

Directions:

1. Pour the black-eyed peas and water into a pot, then cook over medium heat for 25 minutes.
2. Add the beet and carrot to the pot and cook for 10 more minutes. Add more water if necessary.
3. Add the turmeric, cumin, asafetida, parsley, and cayenne pepper to the pot and cook for an additional 6 minutes or until the vegetables are soft. Stir the mixture periodically. Sprinkle with salt, if desired.
4. Drizzle the lime juice on top before serving in a large bowl.

Nutrition:

- Calories: 84
- Fat: 0.7 g
- Carbohydrates: 16.6 g
- Protein: 4.1 g
- Fiber 4.5 g

Peppers and Black Beans with Brown Rice

Preparation Time: 15 minutes
Cooking Time: 20 minutes
Servings: 4
Ingredients:

- 2 jalapeno peppers, diced
- 1 red bell pepper, seeded and diced
- 1 medium yellow onion, peeled and diced
- 2 tablespoons low-sodium vegetable broth
- 1 teaspoon toasted and ground cumin seeds
- 1-½ teaspoons toasted oregano
- 5 garlic cloves, peeled and minced
- 4 cups cooked black beans
- Salt, to taste (optional)
- Ground black pepper, to taste
- 3 cups cooked brown rice
- 1 lime, quartered
- 1 cup chopped cilantro

Directions:

1. Add the jalapeno peppers, bell pepper, and onion to a saucepan and saute for 7 minutes or until the onion is well browned and caramelized.
2. Add vegetable broth, cumin, oregano, and garlic to the pan and saute for 3 minutes or until fragrant.
3. Add the black beans and saute for 10 minutes or until the vegetables are tender. Sprinkle with salt (if desired) and black pepper halfway through.
4. Arrange the brown rice on a platter, then top with the cooked vegetables. Garnish with lime wedges and cilantro before serving.

Nutrition:

- Calories: 426
- Fat: 2.6 g
- Carbohydrates: 82.4 g
- Protein: 20.2 g
- Fiber 19.5 g

Black Lentil Curry

Preparation Time: 30 minutes
Cooking Time: 6 hours and 15 minutes
Servings: 4
Ingredients:

- 1 cup black lentils, rinsed and soaked overnight
- 14 ounces chopped tomatoes
- 2 large white onions, peeled and sliced
- 1-½ teaspoons minced garlic
- 1 teaspoon grated ginger
- 1 red chili

- 1 teaspoon salt
- ¼ teaspoon red chili powder
- 1 teaspoon paprika
- 1 teaspoon ground turmeric
- 2 teaspoons ground cumin
- 2 teaspoons ground coriander
- ½ cup chopped coriander
- 4 ounces vegetarian butter
- 4 fluid ounce water
- 2 fluid ounce vegetarian double cream

Directions:

1. Place a large pan over moderate heat, add butter and let heat until melt. Add the onion and garlic and ginger and cook for 10 to 15 minutes or until onions are caramelized.
2. Then stir in salt, red chili powder, paprika, turmeric, cumin, ground coriander, and water. Transfer this mixture to a 6-quarts slow cooker and add tomatoes and red chili.
3. Drain lentils, add to slow cooker, and stir until just mix. Plugin slow cooker; adjust Cooking Time to 6 hours and let cook on Low heat setting.
4. When the lentils are done, stir in cream and adjust the seasoning. Serve with boiled rice or whole wheat bread.

Nutrition:
- Calories: 299
- Protein: 5.59 g
- Fat: 27.92 g
- Carbohydrates: 9.83 g

Potato Lentil Stew

Preparation Time: 15 minutes
Cooking Time: 30 minutes
Servings: 4
Ingredients:
- 2 sprigs chopped oregano sprigs
- 1 Diced celery stalk
- 1 cup cubed and peeled potato
- 2 sliced carrots
- 1 cup dry lentils
- 1 teaspoon spicy condiment/pepper
- 1 to 1-½ teaspoons seawater salt
- 2 mashed garlic bulbs
- ½ cup diced onion
- 2 tablespoons avocado oil
- 13-½ ounces full-fat coconut milk
- 5 cups vegetable broth, divided
- 2 sprigs chopped tarragon

Directions:

1. Using a big cooking utensil, warm the avocado grease together with putting in seasonings: pepper, salt, garlic bulbs, together with onion. Cook within 3 to 5 minutes, or until the onion has become soft.
2. Mix in the tarragon, oregano, celery, potato, carrots, lentils, and 2-½ cups of vegetable broth. Mix everything together.
3. Enable the casserole to return up to heat and then lower the fire down. Let this cook, stirring often. Add in an extra vegetable broth in half cup portions as needed.
4. Let the stew cook for 20 to 25 minutes, or until the lentils and potatoes are soft. Set the stew off the heat and mix in the coconut milk. Divide into four bowls and enjoy.

Nutrition:
- Calories: 240
- Carbohydrates: 14 g
- Fat: 17 g
- Protein: 6 g

Tex-Mex Tofu & Beans

Preparation Time: 25 minutes
Cooking Time: 12 minutes
Servings: 2
Ingredients:
- 1 cup dry black beans
- 1 cup dry brown rice
- 14 ounces package firm tofu, drained
- 2 tablespoons olive oil
- 1 small purple onion, diced
- 1 medium avocado, pitted, peeled
- 1 garlic clove, minced
- 1 tablespoon lime juice
- 2 teaspoons cumin
- 2 teaspoons paprika
- 1 teaspoon chili powder
- Salt and pepper to taste

Directions:

1. Cut the tofu into ½-inch cubes. Heat the olive oil in a skillet. Put the diced onions and cook until soft, for about 5 minutes.
2. Add the tofu and cook for an additional 2 minutes, flipping the cubes frequently. Meanwhile, cut the avocado into thin slices and set them aside.
3. Lower the heat and add in the garlic, cumin, and cooked black beans. Stir until everything is incorporated thoroughly, and then cook for an additional 5 minutes.

4. Add the remaining spices and lime juice to the mixture in the skillet. Mix thoroughly and remove the skillet from heat.
5. Serve the Tex-Mex tofu and beans with a scoop of rice and garnish with the fresh avocado. Enjoy immediately, or store the rice, avocado, and tofu mixture separately.

Nutrition:
- Calories: 315
- Carbohydrates: 27.8 g
- Fat: 17 g
- Protein: 12.7 g

Quinoa Lentil Burger

Preparation Time: 5 minutes
Cooking Time: 25 minutes
Servings: 4
Ingredients:
- 1 tablespoon plus 2 teaspoons olive oil
- ¼ cup red onion, diced
- 1 cup quinoa, cooked
- 1 cup cooked drained brown lentils
- 1x4 ounces green chilies, diced
- ⅓ cup oats, rolled
- ¼ cup flour
- 2 teaspoons corn starch
- ¼ cup panko breadcrumbs, whole-wheat
- ¼ teaspoon garlic powder
- ½ teaspoon cumin
- 1 teaspoon paprika
- Salt and pepper, to taste
- 2 tablespoons Dijon mustard
- 3 teaspoons honey

Directions:
1. Put 2 teaspoons olive oil into your skillet over medium heat. Add the onion and cook for five minutes until soft. Grab a small bowl and add the honey and Dijon mustard.
2. Grab a large bowl and add the burger ingredients; stir well. Form into 4 patties with your hands. Put a tablespoon of oil into your skillet over medium heat.
3. Add the patties and cook for 10 minutes on each side. Serve with the honey mustard and enjoy!

Nutrition:
- Calories: 268 Carbohydrates: 33 g
- Fat: 8 g Protein: 10 g

Broccoli & Black Beans Stir Fry

Preparation Time: 15 minutes
Cooking Time: 10 minutes
Servings: 6
Ingredients:
- 4 cups broccoli florets
- 2 cups cooked black beans
- 1 tablespoon sesame oil
- 4 teaspoons sesame seeds
- 2 garlic cloves, finely minced
- 2 teaspoons ginger, finely chopped
- A large pinch red chili flake
- A pinch turmeric powders
- Salt to taste
- Lime juice to taste (optional)

Directions:
1. Steam broccoli for 6 minutes. Drain and set aside. Warm the sesame oil in your large frying pan over medium heat.
2. Add sesame seeds, chili flakes, ginger, garlic, turmeric powder, and salt. Saute for a couple of minutes.
3. Add broccoli and black beans and saute until thoroughly heated. Sprinkle lime juice and serve hot.

Nutrition:
- Calories: 306
- Carbohydrates: 8 g
- Fat: 16 g
- Protein: 31 g

Greek-Style Gigante Beans

Preparation Time: 8 hours and 5 minutes
Cooking Time: 10 hours
Servings: 10
Ingredients:
- 12 ounces Gigante beans
- 1 can tomatoes with juice, chopped
- 2 stalks celery, diced
- 1 onion, diced
- 4 garlic cloves, minced
- Salt, to taste

Directions:
1. Soak beans in water for 8 hours. Combine drained beans with the remaining ingredients. Stir, and pour water to cover. Cook for 10 hours on Low. Season with salt, and serve.

Nutrition:
- Calories: 63
- Carbohydrates: 13 g
- Fat: 2 g

- Protein: 4 g

Mexican Lentil Soup

Preparation Time: 5 minutes
Cooking Time: 45 minutes

Servings: 6

Ingredients:

- 2 cups green lentils
- 1 medium red bell pepper, cored, diced
- 1 medium white onion, peeled, diced
- 2 cups diced tomatoes
- 8 ounces diced green chilies
- 2 celery stalks, diced
- 2 medium carrots, peeled, diced
- 1-½ teaspoon minced garlic
- ½ teaspoon salt
- 1 tablespoon cumin
- ¼ teaspoon smoked paprika
- 1 teaspoon oregano
- ⅛ teaspoon hot sauce
- 2 tablespoons olive oil
- 8 cups vegetable broth
- ¼ cup cilantro, for garnish
- 1 avocado, peeled, pitted, diced, for garnish

Directions:

1. Take a large pot over medium heat, add oil, and when hot, add all the vegetables, reserving tomatoes and chilies, and cook for 5 minutes until softened.
2. Then add garlic, stir in oregano, cumin, and paprika, and continue cooking for 1 minute.
3. Add lentils, tomatoes and green chilies, season with salt, pour in the broth, and simmer the soup for 40 minutes until cooked.
4. When done, ladle soup into bowls, top with avocado and cilantro, and serve straight away

Nutrition:

- Calories: 235 Fat: 9 g
- Carbohydrates: 32 g
- Protein: 9 g

Chapter 8:   Snack & Appetizers

Mixed Seed Crackers

Preparation Time: 20 minutes
Cooking Time: 40 minutes
Servings: 30
Ingredients:

- 1 cup boiling water
- ¼ cup coconut oil, melted
- 1 teaspoon salt
- 1 tablespoon psyllium husk powder
- ⅓ cup sesame seeds
- ⅓ cup flaxseed
- ⅓ cup pumpkin seeds, unsalted
- ⅓ cup sunflower seeds, unsalted
- ⅓ cup almond flour

Directions:

1. Set the oven to 300°Fahrenheit. With a fork, combine the almond flour, seeds, psyllium, and salt. Cautiously pour the boiling water and oil into the bowl, using the fork to combine.
2. The mixture should form a gel-like consistency. Line a cookie sheet using a non-stick paper or a similar alternative, and transfer the mixture to the cookie sheet.
3. Using the second sheet of parchment, place it on top of the mixture, and with a rolling pin, roll out the mixture to an even and flat consistency.
4. Remove the top parchment paper then bake within 40 minutes, frequently checking to ensure the seeds do not burn.
5. After 40 minutes, or when the seeds are browning, turn off the oven but leave the crackers inside for further cooking. Once cool, break into pieces and enjoy.

Nutrition:

- Calories: 28 Protein: 0.44 g
- Fat: 2.15 g Carbohydrates: 1.89 g

Crispy Squash Chips

Preparation Time: 10 minutes
Cooking Time: 20 minutes
Servings: 2
Ingredients:

- 1 teaspoon cayenne pepper
- 1 teaspoon cumin
- 1 teaspoon paprika
- 1 tablespoon avocado oil

- 1 medium butternut squash, skinny neck
- Sea salt to taste

Directions:

1. Set the oven to 375°Fahrenheit heat setting. Prepare the butternut squash by removing the top. Using a mandolin, cut the squash into even slices; it is unnecessary to skin the squash.
2. In a big mixing bowl, place your slices of squash and cover with oil, use your hands to mix them well. Ensure all slices are oiled.
3. Line a cookie sheet using parchment paper and spread out your slices, so they do not overlap.
4. In a little bowl, mix together cayenne pepper, paprika, and cumin, then sprinkle the chips over the top. Season with sea salt to taste. Once cool, enjoy alone or with your favorite dip.

Nutrition:

- Calories: 113
- Protein: 3.66 g
- Fat: 10.57 g
- Carbohydrates: 1.6 g

Paprika Nuts

Preparation Time: 15 minutes
Cooking Time: 15 minutes
Servings: 8
Ingredients:

- 1-½ teaspoons smoked paprika
- 1 teaspoon salt
- 2 tablespoons garlic-infused olive oil
- 1 cup cashews
- 1 cup almonds
- 1 cup pecans
- 1 cup walnuts

Directions:

1. Adjust the rack in the middle of your oven. Set the oven to 325°Fahrenheit before you start preparing the ingredients.
2. In a big mixing bowl, toss the nuts. Pour olive oil over the nuts and toss to coat all the nuts.
3. Sprinkle the salt and paprika over the nuts and mix well. If you want more paprika flavor, then add additional paprika.
4. Line a big cookie sheet using parchment and spread the nuts out in one layer. Bake for approximately 15 minutes, then remove from oven and let cool. Enjoy.

Nutrition:

- Calories: 67
- Protein: 1.28 g
- Fat: 2.46 g
- Carbohydrates: 11.29 g

Basil Zoodles and Olives

Preparation Time: 30 minutes
Cooking Time: 4 hours
Servings: 6
Ingredients:

- 1 can black olives pitted
- 1 little container cherry tomatoes, halved
- 4 medium-sized zucchinis

Sauce:

- ½ cup basil leaves, chopped
- ½ teaspoon pink Himalayan salt
- 2 teaspoons nutritional yeast
- 1 tablespoon lemon juice
- ½ cup water
- ¼ cup sunflower seeds, soaked
- ¼ cup cashew nuts, soaked

Directions:

1. Begin by preparing the sunflower seeds and cashews. Place each in a little bowl and cover with water. Allow to soak for 4 hours, then drain and rinse well.
2. Next, place the seeds and cashews into a blender and mix until completely blended. Then add in basil, salt, nutritional yeast, lemon juice, and water. Blend until a smooth sauce is formed.
3. Using a spiralizer, make the zoodles from the zucchini. Place the zoodles in a big serving bowl and then pour the sauce over the top. Stir to combine. Top with cherry tomatoes and olives.
4. Serve and enjoy.

Nutrition:

- Calories: 56 Protein: 3.28 g
- Fat: 1.54 g Carbohydrates: 8.58 g

Roasted Beetroot Noodles

Preparation Time: 15 minutes
Cooking Time: 20 minutes
Servings: 4
Ingredients:

- 1 teaspoon orange zest

- 2 tablespoons parsley, chopped
- 2 tablespoons balsamic vinegar
- 2 tablespoons olive oil
- 2 big beets, peeled and spiraled

Directions:

1. Set the oven to 425°Fahrenheit high-heat settings. In a big bowl, combine the beet noodles, olive oil, and vinegar. Toss until well combined. Season with pepper and salt.
2. Line a big cookie sheet using parchment paper, and spread the noodles out into a single layer. Roast the noodles for 20 minutes.
3. Place into bowls and zest with orange and sprinkle parsley.
4. Gently toss and serve.

Nutrition:

- Calories: 44
- Protein: 2.71 g
- Fat: 1.71 g
- Carbohydrates: 5.02 g

Strawberry Gazpacho

Preparation Time: 15 minutes
Cooking Time: 0 minutes
Servings: 4
Ingredients:

- 3 large avocados, peeled, pitted and chopped
- ⅓ cup fresh cilantro leaves
- 3 cups homemade vegetable broth
- 2 tablespoons fresh lemon juice
- 1 teaspoon ground cumin
- ¼ teaspoon cayenne pepper
- Salt, to taste

Directions:

1. In a blender, add all fixings and pulse until smooth. Transfer the gazpacho into a large bowl. Cover and refrigerate to chill completely before serving.

Nutrition:

- Calories: 227
- Fat: 20.4 g
- Carbohydrates: 9 g
- Protein: 4.5 g

Cauliflower Popcorn

Preparation Time: 10 minutes
Cooking Time: 12 hours
Servings: 2
Ingredients:

- 2 heads cauliflower
- Spicy sauce
- ½ cup filtered water
- ½ teaspoon turmeric
- 1 cup dates
- 2-3 tablespoons nutritional yeast
- ¼ cup sun-dried tomatoes
- 2 tablespoons raw tahini

- 1-2 teaspoons cayenne pepper
- 2 teaspoons onion powder
- 1 tablespoon apple cider vinegar
- 2 teaspoons garlic powder

Directions:

1. Chop the cauliflower into small pieces. Put all the ingredients for the spicy sauce in a blender and create a mixture with a smooth consistency.
2. Coat the cauliflower florets in the sauce. See that each piece is properly covered. Put the spicy florets in a dehydrator tray.
3. Add some salt and your favorite herb if you want. Dehydrate the cauliflower for 12 hours at 115°Fahrenheit. Keep dehydrating until it is crunchy.
4. Enjoy the cauliflower popcorn.

Nutrition:

- Calories: 491
- Protein: 19.97 g
- Fat: 12.84 g
- Carbohydrates: 86.15 g

Hummus Made with Sweet Potato

Preparation Time: 15 minutes
Cooking Time: 55 minutes
Servings: 3-4
Ingredients:

- 2 cups cooked chickpeas
- 2 medium sweet potatoes
- 3 tablespoons tahini
- 3 tablespoons olive oil
- 3 freshly peeled garlic cloves
- Freshly squeezed lemon juice
- Ground sea salt, to taste
- ¼ teaspoon cumin
- Zest from half a lemon
- ½ teaspoon smoked paprika
- 1-½ teaspoons cayenne pepper

Directions:

1. Set the oven to 400°Fahrenheit. Add the sweet potatoes to the middle rack of the oven and bake them for about 45 minutes.
2. Allow the sweet potatoes to cool. Add all the other ingredients in a food processor then blend. After the sweet potatoes have sufficiently cooled down, use a knife to peel off the skin.
3. Add the sweet potatoes to a blender and blend well with the rest of the ingredients. Once you have a potato mash, sprinkle some sesame seeds and cayenne pepper and serve it!

Nutrition:

- Calories: 376
- Protein: 12.02 g
- Fat: 20.14 g
- Carbohydrates: 40.09 g

Avocado Guacamole

Preparation Time: 15 minutes
Cooking Time: 0 minutes
Servings: 4
Ingredients:

- 2 small ripe avocados, peeled, pitted and chopped
- ½ cup fresh cilantro leaves, chopped finely
- 1 tablespoon fresh lime juice
- A pinch freshly ground black pepper

Directions:

1. In a bowl, add all ingredients, and with a fork, mash until well combined.
2. Serve immediately.

Nutrition:

- Calories: 145
- Fat: 13.8 g
- Carbohydrates: 6.2 g
- Protein: 1.4 g

Strawberry Milkshake

Preparation Time: 5 minutes
Cooking Time: 0 minutes
Servings: 1
Ingredients:

- 2 cups hulled strawberries
- 1 cup nondairy milk
- ½ cup plain non-dairy yogurt or canned coconut milk
- 1 tablespoon sugar, maple syrup, or simple syrup (optional)
- Ice cubes, for blending (optional)

Directions:

1. In a blender, combine the strawberries, milk, yogurt, sugar (if using), and ice (if using). Puree until smooth and creamy.

Nutrition:

- Calories: 268
- Protein: 6 g
- Fat: 6 g
- Carbohydrates: 51 g

Peanut Butter–Mocha Energy Bites

Preparation Time: 45 minutes

Cooking Time: 0 minutes
Servings: 12
Ingredients:

- ¼ cup creamy peanut butter
- 2 tablespoons maple syrup or simple syrup
- 1 tablespoon nondairy milk or water, plus more as needed
- 1 to 2 teaspoons instant coffee powder or chopped roasted coffee beans (optional)
- 2 tablespoons sugar
- 2 tablespoons unsweetened cocoa powder
- 1 tablespoon ground flaxseed
- ½ cup cooked quinoa
- 2 tablespoons plant-based protein powder, coconut flour, or ground almonds

Directions:

1. Stir the peanut butter, maple syrup, and milk in a large bowl until smooth. Add the coffee powder (if using), sugar, cocoa powder, and flaxseed stir to combine.
2. Stir in the quinoa and protein powder. Drizzle in another tablespoon of milk to moisten, if needed.
3. Divide the mixture into about 12 portions, and roll each into a small ball. Place them on a plate and refrigerate, if you can, for 30 minutes.
4. They will keep in an airtight container in the refrigerator for up to 1 week. If you don't have a fridge, enjoy them the same day.

Nutrition:

- Calories: 70
- Protein: 3 g
- Fat: 3 g
- Carbohydrates: 8 g

Cinnamon-Lime Sunflower Seeds

Preparation Time: 5 minutes
Cooking Time: 5 minutes
Servings: 8
Ingredients:

- 1 cup sunflower seeds
- 1 tablespoon sugar, maple syrup, or simple syrup
- A pinch salt
- 1 tablespoon freshly squeezed lime juice
- 1 to 2 teaspoons ground cinnamon or pumpkin pie spice

Directions:

1. Put the sunflower seeds in a large skillet, and cook over medium heat, tossing continuously, for 3 to 5 minutes, until lightly browned.
2. Add the sugar and salt, and keep tossing the seeds. Remove from the heat, and add the lime

juice and cinnamon, tossing quickly to coat while the juice sizzles.

Nutrition:

- Calories: 169
- Protein: 5 g
- Fat: 14 g
- Carbohydrates: 8 g

Bruschetta

Preparation Time: 15 minutes
Cooking Time: 5 minutes
Servings: 4
Ingredients:

- 1 tomato, finely diced
- 1 tablespoon chopped onion or scallion
- Salt to taste
- ½ baguette, sliced, or 2 bread slices
- 1 tablespoon olive oil
- Freshly ground black pepper, to taste

Directions:

1. Toss the tomato, onion, and a pinch of salt in a small bowl. Transfer to a strainer, and let drain in the sink or over a bowl for a few minutes while you prep the bread. Toast the bread lightly.
2. Return the drained tomato mixture to the bowl. Drizzle with the olive oil and season to taste with pepper.
3. If using full slices of bread, cut each in half. Scoop the tomato batter on top of the toasts right before serving.

Nutrition:

- Calories: 70
- Protein: 2 g
- Fat: 4 g
- Carbohydrates: 7 g

Cheese Cucumber Bites

Preparation Time: 10 minutes
Cooking Time: 0 minutes
Servings: 8
Ingredients:

- 4 large cucumbers
- 1 cup raw sunflower seeds
- ½ teaspoon salt
- 2 tablespoons raw red onion, chopped
- 1 handful fresh chives, chopped
- 1 clove fresh garlic, chopped
- 2 tablespoons nutritional yeast
- 2 tablespoons fresh lemon juice
- ½ cup water

Directions:

1. Start by blending sunflower seeds with salt in a food processor for 20 seconds. Toss in remaining ingredients except for the cucumber and chives and process until smooth.
2. Slice the cucumber into 1.5-inch-thick rounds. Top each slice with sunflower mixture. Garnish with sumac and chives.
3. Serve.

Nutrition:
- Calories: 211 Fat: 25.5 g
- Carbohydrates: 32.4 g
- Protein: 1.4 g

Mango Sticky Rice

Preparation Time: 15 minutes
Cooking Time: 20 minutes
Servings: 3
Ingredients:
- ½ cup sugar
- 1 mango, sliced
- 14 ounces coconut milk, canned
- ½ cup basmati rice

Directions:
1. Cook your rice per package instructions, and add half of your sugar. When cooking your rice, substitute half of your water for half of your coconut milk.
2. Boil your remaining coconut milk in a saucepan with your remaining sugar. Boil on high heat until it's thick, and then add in your mango slices.

Nutrition:
- Calories: 571
- Protein: 6 g
- Fat: 29.6 g
- Carbohydrates: 77.6 g

Green Chips

Preparation Time: 15 minutes
Cooking Time: 10-20 minutes
Servings: 2
Ingredients:
- 2 or 3 large green leaves or 5 or 6 small leaves kale, cabbage, collards, orchard, washed, dried, stemmed, and torn into small pieces
- 1 tablespoon olive oil
- 1 tablespoon nutritional yeast (optional)
- 1 teaspoon onion powder (optional)
- A pinch salt

Directions:
1. Preheat the oven to 300°Fahrenheit. Put the greens on a rimmed baking sheet, and sprinkle

with the olive oil, nutritional yeast (if using), onion powder (if using), and salt.
2. Massage the spices into the leaves. Spread the leaves out in a single layer so they dry evenly. Bake for 10 to 20 minutes, until the greens are crispy and dry.
3. Remove the greens from the oven, and let them sit for a few minutes to cool before serving. Store in an airtight container, though it's best to bake and enjoy them the same day.

Nutrition:
- Calories: 93
- Protein: 2 g
- Fat: 7 g
- Carbohydrates: 7 g

Crispy Honey Pecans

Preparation Time: 2 hours and 15 minutes
Cooking Time: 3 hours
Servings: 4
Ingredients:
- 16 ounces pecan halves
- 4 tablespoons coconut butter melted
- 4 to 5 tablespoons honey strained
- ¼ teaspoon ground ginger
- ¼ teaspoon ground allspice
- 1-½ teaspoons ground cinnamon

Directions:
1. Add pecans and melted coconut butter into your 4-quart Slow Cooker. Stir until combined well. Add in honey and stir well.
2. In a bowl, combine spices and sprinkle over nuts; stir lightly. Cook on low uncovered for about 2 to 3 hours or until nuts is crispy. Serve cold.

Nutrition:
- Calories: 220
- Carbohydrates: 29 g
- Fat: 14 g
- Protein: 2 g

Crunchy Fried Pickles

Preparation Time: 10 minutes
Cooking Time: 5 minutes
Servings: 6
Ingredients:
- ½ cup vegetable oil for frying
- 1 cup all-purpose flour
- 1 cup plain breadcrumbs
- A pinch salt and pepper
- 30 pickle chips (cucumber, dill)

Directions:

1. Heat oil in a large frying skillet over medium-high heat. Stir the flour, breadcrumbs, and salt, and pepper in a shallow bowl.
2. Dredge the pickles in the flour/breadcrumbs mixture to coat completely. Fry in batches until golden brown on all sides, 2 to 3 minutes in total. Drain on paper towels and serve.

Nutrition:
- Calories: 287
- Carbohydrates: 28 g
- Fat: 19 g
- Protein: 4 g

Lime and Chili Carrots Noodles

Preparation Time: 10 minutes
Cooking Time: 0 minutes
Servings: 4
Ingredients:
- ½ teaspoon black pepper
- ½ teaspoon salt
- 2 tablespoons coconut oil
- ¼ cup coriander, finely chopped
- 2 jalapeno chilis
- 1 tablespoon lime juice
- 2 carrots, peeled and spiralized

Directions:
1. In a little bowl, combine jalapeno, lime juice, and coconut oil to form a sauce. In a big bowl, place the carrot noodles and pour dressing over the top.
2. Toss to ensure the dressing fully coats the noodles. Season with pepper and salt.
3. Serve and enjoy.

Nutrition:
- Calories: 93 Protein: 1.92 g
- Fat: 8.4 g Carbohydrates: 3.28 g

Sweet Potato Tots

Preparation Time: 5 minutes
Cooking Time: 30 minutes
Servings: 25
Ingredients:
- 2 cups sweet potato puree
- ½ teaspoon ground cumin
- ½ teaspoon salt
- ½ teaspoon ground coriander
- ½ cup panko breadcrumbs
- Olive oil spray just enough to coat the pan

Directions:
1. Switch on the Air Fryer, insert the fryer basket, then shut it with the lid. Set the frying temperature to 390°Fahrenheit, and let it preheat for 5 minutes.

2. Meanwhile, take a large bowl and place all the ingredients in it. Stir until well combined, and then shape the mixture into twenty-five tots, each about 1 tablespoon.
3. Open the preheated fryer and place sweet potato tots in it in a single layer. Spray with olive oil, close the lid and cook for 14 minutes until golden brown and cooked, turning and spraying with oil halfway.
4. When done, the Air Fryer will beep. Then open the lid, transfer tots to a dish and cover with foil to keep them warm. Cook remaining tots in the same manner and then serve straight away.

Nutrition:
- Calories: 26
- Fat: 0.2 g
- Carbohydrates: 6 g
- Proteins 0 g

Avocado Fries

Preparation Time: 5 minutes
Cooking Time: 10 minutes
Servings: 4
Ingredients:
- 1 medium avocado, peeled, pitted, sliced
- ½ teaspoon salt
- ½ cup panko breadcrumbs
- ¼ cup chickpeas liquid
- Olive oil spray

Directions:
1. Switch on the Air Fryer and insert the fryer basket. Then shut it with the lid. Set the frying temperature to 390°Fahrenheit, and let it preheat for 5 minutes.
2. Meanwhile, take a shallow bowl and place breadcrumbs in it. Season with salt, and stir until combined.
3. Take another shallow bowl and pour in chickpeas liquid. Dip avocado slices and dredge into breadcrumbs mixture until coated.
4. Open the preheated fryer and place avocado slices in it in a single layer. Spray with olive oil, close the lid and cook for 10 minutes until golden brown and cooked, shaking, and spraying with oil halfway.
5. When done, the Air Fryer will beep. Then open the lid and transfer avocado fries to a dish. Serve straight away.

Nutrition:
- Calories: 132
- Protein: 4 g
- Carbohydrates: 7 g
- Fat: 11 g

Italian Tomato Snack

Preparation Time: 10 minutes
Cooking Time: 60 minutes
Servings: 6
Ingredients:

- 50 ounces canned tomatoes, drained
- A pinch salt and black pepper
- ¼ cup extra virgin olive oil
- 15 basil leaves, sliced
- 1 tablespoon burgundy or merlot wine vinegar
- A pinch stevia
- 10 baguette pieces, toasted

Directions:

1. Spread the tomatoes on the lined baking sheet. Drizzle half of the oil; season with salt and pepper and bake them at 300°Fahrenheit for one hour.
2. Slice the tomatoes into cubes and put them inside a bowl with the oil, basil, vinegar and stevia and toss. Split the tomatoes on each baguette slice and serve as a snack.

Nutrition:

- Calories: 191
- Fat: 4 g
- Carbohydrates: 9 g
- Protein: 7 g

Easy Dried Grapes

Preparation Time: 5 minutes
Cooking Time: 4 hours
Servings: 10
Ingredients:

- 3 bunches seedless grapes
- A drizzle vegetable oil

Directions:

1. Spread the grapes over a lined baking sheet and drizzle the oil. Toss and bake at 225°Fahrenheit for 4 hours.
2. Separate the grapes into bowls and serve.

Nutrition:

- Calories: 131
- Fat: 1 g
- Protein: 3 g
- Carbohydrates: 5 g

Rosemary and Lemon Zest Popcorn

Preparation Time: 10 minutes
Cooking Time: 0 minutes
Servings: 2
Ingredients:

- ⅓ cup popcorn kernels
- 2 tablespoons vegan butter, melted
- 1 tablespoon chopped rosemary
- 1 teaspoon lemon zest
- ¼ teaspoon salt

Directions:

1. Pop the kernels, and when done, transfer them into a large bowl. Drizzle butter over the popcorns, sprinkle with salt, lemon zest, and rosemary, and then toss until combined.
2. Serve straight away.

Nutrition:

- Calories: 201 Protein: 3 g
- Carbohydrates: 25 g Fat: 10 g

Strawberry Avocado Toast

Preparation Time: 5 minutes
Cooking Time: 0 minutes
Servings: 4
Ingredients:

- 1 avocado, peeled, pitted, and quartered
- 4 whole-wheat bread slices, toasted
- 4 ripe strawberries, cut into ¼-inch slices
- 1 tablespoon balsamic glaze or reduction

Directions:

1. Mash one-quarter of your avocado on a slice of toast. Put one-quarter of the strawberry slices over your avocado, then finish with a drizzle of balsamic glaze.
2. Repeat with the remaining fixings, and serve.

Nutrition:

- Calories: 150 Fat: 8 g
- Carbohydrates: 17 g Protein: 5 g

Strawberry Watermelon Ice Pops

Preparation Time: 6 hours and 5 minutes
Cooking Time: 0 minutes
Servings: 6
Ingredients:

- 4 cups diced watermelon
- 4 strawberries, tops removed
- 2 tablespoons freshly squeezed lime juice

Directions:

1. Combine the watermelon, strawberries, and lime juice in a blender. Blend within 1 to 2 minutes, or until well combined.
2. Pour evenly into 6 ice-pop molds, insert ice-pop sticks, and freeze for at least 6 hours before serving.

Nutrition:

- Calories: 61
- Fat: 0 g
- Carbohydrates: 15 g

- Protein: 1 g

Seed Bars

Preparation Time: 15 minutes
Cooking Time: 15 minutes
Servings: 10
Ingredients:

- 1-¼ cups creamy salted peanut butter
- 5 Medjool dates, pitted
- ½ cup unsweetened vegan protein powder
- ⅔ cup hemp seeds
- ⅓ cup chia seeds

Directions:

1. Line a loaf pan with parchment paper. Set aside. In a food processor, add the peanut butter and dates and pulse until well combined.
2. Add the protein powder, hemp seeds, and chia seeds and pulse until well combined. Now, place the mixture into the prepared loaf pan, and with the back of a spoon, smooth the top surface.
3. Freeze for at least 10–15 minutes, or until set. Cut into 10 equal-sized bars and serve.

Nutrition:

- Calories: 308
- Fat: 21 g
- Carbohydrates: 17 g
- Protein: 16 g

Chocolate Protein: Bites

Preparation Time: 10 minutes
Cooking Time: 20 minutes
Servings: 12
Ingredients:

- ½ cup chocolate protein powder
- 1 avocado, medium
- 1 tablespoon chocolate chips
- 1 tablespoon almond butter
- 1 tablespoon cocoa powder
- 1 teaspoon vanilla extract
- A pinch salt

Directions:

1. Begin by blending avocado, almond butter, vanilla extract, and salt in a high-speed blender until you get a smooth mixture.
2. Next, spoon in the protein powder, cocoa powder, and chocolate chips to the blender. Blend again until you get a smooth dough-like consistency mixture.
3. Now, check for seasoning and add more sweetness if needed. Finally, with the help of a scooper, scoop out dough to make small balls.

Nutrition:

- Calories: 46

- Fat: 2 g
- Carbohydrates: 2 g
- Protein: 2 g

Lentil Cakes

Preparation Time: 10 minutes
Cooking Time: 10 minutes
Servings: 8
Ingredients:

- 2 teaspoons basil, dried
- 1 cup chopped yellow onion
- 1 cup leeks, chopped
- 1 cup canned red lentils, drained and rinsed
- 1 teaspoon coriander, ground
- ¼ cup chopped parsley
- 1 tablespoon curry powder
- ¼ cup chopped cilantro
- 2 tablespoons coconut flour
- 1 tablespoon olive oil

Directions:

1. Put the lentils in your bowl and mash them well using a potato masher. Add the basil, onion, and the other ingredients except for the oil and stir. Shape medium cakes out of this mix.
2. Warm up a pan with the oil over medium-high heat. Add the cakes and cook them for about 5 minutes on each side.
3. Serve warm.

Nutrition:

- Calories: 142 Fat: 4 g
- Carbohydrates: 8 g Protein: 4.4 g

Balsamic Green Beans Bowls

Preparation Time: 10 minutes
Cooking Time: 25 minutes
Servings: 4
Ingredients:

- 1-pound green beans, trimmed and halved
- A pinch salt and black pepper
- 1 teaspoon turmeric powder
- 1 teaspoon sweet paprika
- 4 tablespoons balsamic vinegar
- 1 teaspoon Italian seasoning

Directions:

1. Spread the green beans on a lined baking sheet. Add the rest of the ingredients. Toss and bake at 430°Fahrenheit for 25 minutes.
2. Serve as a snack.

Nutrition:

- Calories: 210
- Fat: 5.5 g
- Carbohydrates: 11 g

- Protein: 6.3 g

Kale Bowls

Preparation Time: 10 minutes
Cooking Time: 10 minutes
Servings: 4
Ingredients:

- 2 tablespoons almonds, chopped
- 2 tablespoons walnuts, chopped
- 2 bunches kale, trimmed and roughly chopped
- 1 cup cherry tomatoes, halved
- Salt and black pepper to taste
- 2 tablespoons avocado oil
- 1 lemon juice
- $^2/_3$ cup jarred roasted peppers
- 1 teaspoon Italian seasoning
- ¼ teaspoon chili powder

Directions:

1. Warm up a pan with the oil over medium heat. Add kale and cook for 5 minutes.
2. Add the rest of the ingredients. Toss; cook for 5 minutes more. Divide into bowls and serve.

Nutrition:

- Calories: 143
- Fat: 5.9 g
- Carbohydrates: 9 g
- Protein: 7 g

Green Bean Fries

Preparation Time: 10 minutes
Cooking Time: 8 hours
Servings: 8
Ingredients:

- $^1/_3$ cup avocado oil
- 5 pounds green beans, trimmed
- Salt and black pepper to taste
- 1 teaspoon garlic powder
- 1 teaspoon onion powder

- 1 teaspoon turmeric powder
- 1 teaspoon oregano, dried
- 1 teaspoon mint, dried

Directions:

1. Mix the green beans with the oil, salt, pepper, and the other ingredients in a bowl and toss well.
2. Put the green beans in your dehydrator and dry them for 8 hours at 135°Fahrenheit.
3. Serve cold as a snack.

Nutrition:

- Calories: 100
- Fat: 12 g
- Carbohydrates: 8 g
- Protein: 5 g

Seed and Apricot Bowls

Preparation Time: 10 minutes
Cooking Time: 10 minutes
Servings: 4
Ingredients:

- 6 ounces apricots, dried
- 1 cup sunflower seeds
- 2 tablespoons coconut, shredded
- 1 tablespoon sesame seeds
- 1 tablespoon avocado oil
- 3 tablespoons hemp seeds
- 1 tablespoon chia seeds

Directions:

1. Spread the apricots, seeds, and the other ingredients on a lined baking sheet. Toss and cook at 430°Fahrenheit for 10 minutes.
2. Cool down, divide into bowls and serve as a snack.

Nutrition:

- Calories: 200
- Fat: 4.3 g
- Carbohydrates: 8 g
- Protein: 5 g

Chapter 9:   Sauces, Dips & Condiments

Tomato and Avocado Salsa

Preparation Time: 10 minutes
Cooking Time: 0 minutes
Servings: 6
Ingredients:

- 3 cups chopped tomatoes
- 1 cup avocado, peeled, pitted and chopped
- 1 tablespoon black olives, pitted and sliced
- 1 red onion, chopped
- 2 teaspoons capers
- 3 garlic cloves, minced
- 2 teaspoons balsamic vinegar
- 1 tablespoon chopped basil
- A pinch salt and black pepper

Directions:

1. Mix the tomatoes with the avocado, olives, and the other ingredients in a bowl and toss.
2. Serve.

Nutrition:

- Calories: 201
- Fat: 4.9 g
- Carbohydrates: 8 g
- Protein: 6 g

Hearts of Palm & Cheese Dip

Preparation Time: 15 minutes
Cooking Time: 25 minutes
Servings: 9
Ingredients:

- ¼ cup mayonnaise
- ¼ cup parmesan cheese, for topping
- ½ cup parmesan cheese, shredded
- 1 (14 ounces) can heart palm, drained
- 2 large organic eggs, separate 1 egg
- 2 tablespoons Italian seasoning
- 3 stalks green onions, chopped

Directions:

1. Oil a small baking dish with cooking spray and preheat oven to 350°Fahrenheit. In a food processor, add hearts of palm, mayo, parmesan cheese, seasoning, and green onions. Process until chopped thoroughly.
2. Add 1 egg yolk and one whole egg. Pulse four times. Pour mixture into prepared dish. Pop in the oven and bake within 20 minutes.
3. Remove from oven and mix. Top with cheese. Return to oven and broil until tops are golden brown, around 2 to 3 minutes.

Nutrition:

- Calories: 74
- Protein: 4.9 g
- Carbohydrates: 4.2 g
- Fat: 9.2 g

5-Layer Dip

Preparation Time: 15 minutes
Cooking Time: 0 minutes
Servings: 6
Ingredients:

- 1-½ cups refried beans
- 1 cup loaded guacamole
- 1 cup sour cream
- ½ cup chopped pitted olives
- 2 or 3 tomatoes, diced
- ¼ cup salsa
- ½ cup grated vegan cheese (optional)
- Tortilla chips, for serving

Directions:

1. Spread the refried beans in an 8-inch baking dish, followed by guacamole, sour cream, and olives.
2. In a small bowl, stir together the tomatoes and salsa, and spread this mixture over the top of the dip. Sprinkle on the cheese (if using), and serve with tortilla chips for dipping.

Nutrition:

- Calories: 329 Protein: 8 g
- Fat: 17 g
- Carbohydrates: 38 g

Loaded Guacamole

Preparation Time: 15 minutes

Cooking Time: 0 minutes
Servings: 2
Ingredients:

- 1 avocado, halved and pitted
- 1 tomato, diced small
- 1 scallion, white and light green parts only, sliced
- 1 garlic clove, minced
- 2 tablespoons freshly squeezed lime juice
- A pinch salt
- A pinch freshly ground black pepper
- A pinch red pepper flakes (optional)
- Tortilla chips (optional, for serving)

Directions:

1. Spoon the avocado flesh into your medium bowl, and mash it with a fork. Stir in the tomato, scallion, garlic, lime juice, salt, pepper, and red pepper flakes (if using).
2. Enjoy this with tortilla chips, if you like.

Nutrition:

- Calories: 74
- Protein: 1 g
- Fat: 6 g
- Carbohydrates: 7 g

Beans with Sesame Hummus

Preparation Time: 10 minutes
Cooking Time: 0 minutes
Servings: 6
Ingredients:

- 4 tablespoon sesame oil
- 2 garlic cloves finely sliced
- 1 can (15 ounces) cannellini beans, drained
- 4 tablespoons sesame paste
- 2 tablespoons lemon juice freshly squeezed
- ¼ teaspoon red pepper flakes
- 2 tablespoons fresh basil finely chopped
- 2 tablespoons fresh parsley finely chopped
- Sea salt to taste

Directions:

1. Place all ingredients in your food processor. Process until all ingredients are combined well and smooth.
2. Transfer mixture into a bowl and refrigerate until servings.

Nutrition:

- Calories: 80
- Carbohydrates: 5 g
- Fat: 6 g

- Protein: 2 g

Beans and Squash Dip

Preparation Time: 10 minutes
Cooking Time: 6 hours
Servings: 4
Ingredients:

- ½ cup butternut squash, peeled and cubed
- ½ cup canned white beans, drained
- 1 tablespoon water
- 2 tablespoons coconut milk
- ½ teaspoon rosemary, dried
- ½ teaspoon sage, dried
- A pinch salt and black pepper

Directions:

1. In a slow cooker, mix beans with squash, water, coconut milk, sage, rosemary, salt and pepper, toss, cover and cook on Low for 6 hours.
2. Blend using an immersion blender, divide into bowls and serve cold.

Nutrition:

- Calories: 182
- Fat: 5 g
- Carbohydrates: 12 g
- Protein: 4 g

Pea Dip

Preparation Time: 10 minutes
Cooking Time: 0 minutes
Servings: 8
Ingredients:

- 2 cups canned black-eyed peas, drained and rinsed
- ½ teaspoon chili powder
- ½ cup coconut cream
- A pinch salt and black pepper
- ½ teaspoon garlic powder
- 1 teaspoon Italian seasoning
- ½ teaspoon chili sauce
- 1 teaspoon hot paprika

Directions:

1. In a blender, mix the peas with the chili powder, cream, and the other ingredients, blend and serve.

Nutrition:

- Calories: 127
- Fat: 5 g
- Carbohydrates: 18 g
- Protein: 8 g

Mushrooms Salsa

Preparation Time: 10 minutes
Cooking Time: 12 minutes
Servings: 4
Ingredients:

- 1 tablespoon olive oil
- 1 cup cherry tomatoes, halved
- 1 avocado, peeled, pitted and cubed
- 1 tablespoon chives, chopped
- 1 small yellow onion, chopped
- 2 pounds button mushrooms, sliced
- 3 garlic cloves, minced
- 2 cups chopped spinach
- Salt and black pepper totaste
- ¼ cup chopped parsley

Directions:

1. Warm-up a pan with the oil over medium heat. Add the garlic and onion then cook for 2 minutes.
2. Add the mushrooms and the other ingredients. Cook for 10 minutes more; divide into bowls and serve.

Nutrition:

- Calories: 240
- Fat: 8 g
- Carbohydrates: 10.1 g
- Protein: 6.9 g

Tahini Dip

Preparation Time: 10 minutes
Cooking Time: 0 minutes
Servings: 6
Ingredients:

- 1 cup tahini sesame seed paste
- ½ cup coconut cream
- Salt and black pepper to taste
- ½ cup lemon juice
- 1 tablespoon chopped cilantro
- 1 tablespoon chopped chives, chopped
- 1 teaspoon curry powder
- ½ teaspoon ground cumin
- 3 garlic cloves, chopped

Directions:

1. In a blender, mix the tahini paste with the cream and the other ingredients. Blend well, divide into bowls and serve.

Nutrition:

- Calories: 220
- Fat: 12 g
- Carbohydrates: 11 g
- Protein: 7.1 g

Eggplant Spread

Preparation Time: 10 minutes
Cooking Time: 0 minutes
Servings: 6
Ingredients:

- 2 pounds eggplant, baked, peeled and chopped
- A pinch salt and black pepper
- 4 tablespoons avocado oil
- 4 garlic cloves, chopped
- 1 lemon juice
- 1 lemon zest, grated
- 1 teaspoon oregano, dried
- 1 teaspoon basil, dried
- ¼ cup black olives, pitted
- 1 tablespoon sesame paste

Directions:

1. In a blender, mix the eggplant with salt, pepper the oil, and the other ingredients. Blend well and serve.

Nutrition:

- Calories: 215 Fat: 11 g
- Carbohydrates: 8 g Protein: 7.6 g

Coconut Spread

Preparation Time: 10 minutes
Cooking Time: 0 minutes
Servings: 6
Ingredients:

- 2 garlic cloves, minced
- 1 lime juice
- 1-½ cups coconut cream
- 1 tablespoon Italian seasoning
- 4 spring onions, chopped
- A pinch salt and black pepper
- 1 teaspoon oregano, dried
- 1 teaspoon mint, dried

Directions:

1. In a blender, mix the coconut cream with the garlic, lime juice, and the other ingredients. Blend well and serve.

Nutrition:

- Calories: 210
- Fat: 6.7 g
- Carbohydrates: 8 g
- Protein: 5 g

Mushroom Dip

Preparation Time: 10 minutes
Cooking Time: 20 minutes
Servings: 4
Ingredients:

- ¼ cup coconut cream
- 1 teaspoon garlic powder
- 1 teaspoon chili powder
- 1 tablespoon olive oil
- 1 teaspoon oregano, dried
- 1 small yellow onion, chopped
- 24 ounces white mushroom caps
- Salt and black pepper to taste
- 1 teaspoon curry powder

Directions:
1. Heat up a pan with the oil over medium heat. Add the onion, oregano, chili, curry and garlic then cook for 5 minutes. Add the mushrooms and cook for 5 minutes more.
2. Add the rest of the ingredients and cook the mix for 10 minutes. Cool down a bit; blend with an immersion blender and serve as a party dip.

Nutrition:
- Calories: 224
- Fat: 11.4 g
- Carbohydrates: 7 g
- Protein: 11 g

Mango Salsa

Preparation Time: 10 minutes
Cooking Time: 0 minutes
Servings: 4
Ingredients:
- 2 cups cubed mango
- ¼ cup chopped chives
- 1 teaspoon mint, dried
- 1 teaspoon coriander, ground
- 1 tablespoon cilantro, chopped
- ½ cup red bell pepper, minced
- ½ cup chopped red onion
- 2 tablespoons olive oil
- Salt and black pepper to taste
- 1 lime juice
- A pinch red pepper flakes

Directions:
1. In a bowl, mix the mango with the chives, mint, and the other ingredients. Toss and serve.

Nutrition:
- Calories: 100 Fat: 3 g
- Carbohydrates: 8 g Protein: 9 g

Avocado Dip

Preparation Time: 10 minutes
Cooking Time: 0 minutes
Servings: 4
Ingredients:

- 2 avocados, peeled, pitted, chopped
- Salt and black pepper to taste
- 1 tablespoon olive oil
- 1 teaspoon mint, dried
- 1 teaspoon curry powder
- 1 tablespoon green curry paste
- 4 garlic cloves, chopped
- ½ cup tahini
- 2 tablespoons lemon juice

Directions:
1. In a blender, mix the avocado with salt, pepper, oil, and the other ingredients.
2. Pulse until smooth then divide into bowls and serve as a snack.

Nutrition:
- Calories: 200 Fat: 6.3 g
- Carbohydrates: 9 g
- Protein: 7.6 g

Powerful Peas & Lentils Dip

Preparation Time: 10 minutes
Cooking Time: 0 minutes
Servings: 4
Ingredients:
- 4 cups frozen peas
- 2 cup green lentils cooked
- 1 piece grated ginger
- ½ cup fresh basil chopped
- 1 cup ground almonds
- ½ lime juice
- A pinch salt
- 4 tablespoons sesame oil
- ¼ cup sesame seeds

Directions:
1. Place all fixings in a food processor or a blender. Blend until all ingredients combined well.
2. Keep refrigerated in an airtight container for up to 4 days.

Nutrition:
- Calories: 160 Carbohydrates: 31 g
- Fat: 1 g Protein: 7 g

Honey Peanut Butter

Preparation Time: 10 minutes
Cooking Time: 0 minutes
Servings: 6
Ingredients:
- 1 cup peanut butter

- ¾ cup honey extracted
- ½ cup ground peanuts
- 1 teaspoon ground cinnamon

Directions:
1. Add all ingredients into your fast-speed blender, and mix until smooth.
2. Keep refrigerated.

Nutrition:
- Calories: 180
- Carbohydrates: 10 g
- Fat: 14 g
- Protein: 6 g

Spinach Spread

Preparation Time: 10 minutes
Cooking Time: 0 minutes
Servings: 5
Ingredients:
- 4 cups spinach, chopped
- ¼ cup olive oil
- Salt and black pepper to taste
- 4 garlic cloves, minced
- ¾ cup tahini
- ½ cup lime juice
- 1 lime zest, grated
- 1 tablespoon oregano, chopped
- 1 tablespoon chives, chopped

Directions:
1. In your blender, mix the spinach with the oil and the other ingredients. Pulse well, and serve as a party spread.

Nutrition:
- Calories: 110
- Fat: 5.1 g
- Carbohydrates: 6.2 g
- Protein: 3.3 g

Kale Spread

Preparation Time: 10 minutes
Cooking Time: 0 minutes
Servings: 2
Ingredients:
- 3 cups kale, chopped
- 3 tablespoons tomato sauce
- ¼ cup avocado mayonnaise
- Salt and black pepper to taste
- 1 teaspoon mint, chopped
- 1 teaspoon turmeric powder
- ½ teaspoon garlic powder

Directions:
1. In a blender, mix the kale with the tomato sauce and the other ingredients. Blend well and serve.

Nutrition:
- Calories: 100 Fat: 12 g
- Carbohydrates: 1 g
- Protein: 6 g

Keto Caramel Sauce

Preparation Time: 10 minutes
Cooking Time: 35 minutes
Servings: 8
Ingredients:
- ½ cup raw cashews
- ½ cup coconut cream, melted
- 10 drops liquid stevia
- 2 tablespoons vegan butter
- 3 teaspoons vanilla extract
- A pinch salt

Directions:
1. Preheat your oven to 325°Fahrenheit.
2. Place nuts on a greased baking tray and toast for 20 minutes or until lightly golden and crunchy.
3. Allow the nuts to cool slightly; then add to a food processor and blend to slightly lumpy consistency.
4. Add remaining ingredients and blend until a smooth and creamy consistency is achieved. Do not over blend or the coconut cream will become separated from the rest of the ingredients.
5. Can be stored in a glass, airtight container in the refrigerator if not being served immediately. To reheat the caramel to make it more flowable, add to a saucepan and gently warm on low heat. Can be served with your favorite keto vegan treats such as ice cream.

Nutrition:
- Fat: 9.8 g
- Cholesterol 0 mg
- Sodium 29 mg
- Carbohydrates: 4.6 g

Pecan Butter

Preparation Time: 10 minutes
Cooking Time: 10 minutes
Servings: 8
Ingredients:
- 3 cups pecans, soaked well for at least 3 hours, rinsed, strained and dried

Directions:
1. Add the pecans to a food processor and blend until a smooth and creamy consistency is achieved. Scrape down the sides of the bowl when necessary.
2. Transfer to a Mason jar and store in the refrigerator. Can be stored in the refrigerator for

several months. Makes a great spread on toast and sandwiches and a great fruit and veggie dip.

Nutrition:
- Fat: 25 g Cholesterol 0 mg
- Sodium 0 mg
- Carbohydrates: 5 g

Keto Vegan Ranch Dressing

Preparation Time: 5 minutes
Cooking Time: 10 minutes
Servings: 3
Ingredients:
- 1 cup vegan mayonnaise
- 1-½ cups coconut milk
- 2 scallions
- 2 garlic cloves, peeled
- 1 cup fresh dill
- 1 teaspoon garlic powder
- Salt and pepper to taste

Directions:
1. Add scallion, fresh dill, and garlic cloves to a food processor and pulse until finely chopped.
2. Add the rest of the ingredients and blend until a smooth, creamy consistency is achieved. Makes a great creamy salad dressing.
3. Store in the refrigerator.

Nutrition:
- Fat: 11.9 g
- Cholesterol 0 mg
- Sodium 50 mg
- Fiber 4 g

Cauliflower Hummus

Preparation Time: 10 minutes
Cooking Time: 20 minutes
Servings: 7
Ingredients:
- 1 large head cauliflower
- 1 tablespoon almond butter
- 1 garlic clove, finely chopped
- 1 tablespoon lemon juice
- 2 teaspoons olive oil
- ¼ teaspoon cumin
- Salt and pepper to taste

Directions:
1. Cut cauliflower into florets and place in a large microwave-safe bowl. Microwave for 10 minutes on high heat or until completely cooked through.
2. Transfer cauliflower florets to a food processor. Add the rest of the ingredients

3. Blend until a smooth, creamy consistency is reached. Can be stored in the refrigerator in an airtight container for up to 5 days. Makes a great dip for fruits and veggies.

Nutrition:
- Fat: 2.7 g
- Cholesterol 0 mg
- Sodium 12 mg
- Carbohydrates: 2.7 g

Healthier Guacamole

Preparation Time: 10 minutes
Cooking Time: 10 minutes
Servings: 4
Ingredients:
- ¾ cup crumbled tofu
- 2 avocados, peeled and pitted, divided
- 1 teaspoon salt
- 1 teaspoon minced garlic
- A pinch cayenne pepper (optional)

Directions:
1. Prepare a food processor then put one avocado and tofu in it then blend well until it becomes smooth. Combine salt, lime juice, and the left avocado in a bowl.
2. Add in the garlic, tomatoes, cilantro, onion, and tofu-avocado mixture. Put in cayenne pepper.
3. Let it chill in the refrigerator for 1 hour to enhance the flavor or you can serve it right away.

Nutrition:
- Calories: 534 Fat: 5 g Carbohydrates: 23 g
- Protein: 11 g

Chocolate Coconut Butter

Preparation Time: 10 minutes
Cooking Time: 20 minutes
Servings: 20
Ingredients:
- ½ pound unsweetened shredded coconut
- 3 tablespoons cocoa butter
- ⅛ teaspoon salt

Directions:
1. Preheat your oven to 350°Fahrenheit.
2. Place shredded coconut on a greased baking sheet. Spread out into a thin, even layer.
3. Bake for up to 15 minutes or until the coconut flakes are golden brown. Stir the coconut shreds every 3 minutes and watch them closely because they burn very easily and quickly.
4. Allow the coconut flakes to cool for 15 minutes.

5. Add coconut flakes to a food processor and blend until smooth and creamy.
6. Adding cocoa butter and salt and blend to mix well. Pour into an airtight jar and seal the lid. The consistency will thicken up as the butter cools. The oil may separate and float to the top of the container as the butter cools.
7. Simply reheat a portion in the microwave just before using. Can be stored for up to a whole year at room temperature!

Nutrition:
- Fat: 17.4 g Cholesterol 0 mg
- Sodium 17 mg Carbohydrates: 0.9 g
- Fiber 0.6 g Protein: 0.3 g

Orange Dill Butter

Preparation Time: 10 minutes
Cooking Time: 15 minutes
Servings: 12
Ingredients:
- ½ cup vegan butter
- 2 tablespoons fresh dill, finely chopped
- 2 tablespoons orange zest
- 1 teaspoon salt

Directions:
1. Add 4 cups of water to a small pot and bring to a boil over high heat. Reduce heat to low and allow water to simmer.
2. Add vegan butter to a glass Mason jar and screw on the lid loosely.
3. Place Mason jar in the boiling water. Ensure the jar does not get submerged or over-turn.
4. Allow the butter to melt and add the remaining ingredients.
5. Remove the Mason jar from the pot and allow it to cool until the mixture becomes partially solidified.
6. Can be used alongside your favorite veggies to infuse them with flavor and fat. Can be stored in the refrigerator for up to 2 weeks.

Nutrition:
- Fat: 1.5 g
- Cholesterol 0 mg
- Sodium 199 mg
- Carbohydrates: 1 g
- Fiber 0.3 g
- Protein: 0.1 g

Spiced Almond Butter

Preparation Time: 10 minutes
Cooking Time: 5 minutes
Servings: 10
Ingredients:
- 2 cups raw almond

- $1/8$ teaspoon allspice
- $1/8$ teaspoon cinnamon
- $1/8$ teaspoon cardamom
- $1/8$ teaspoon ground ginger
- $1/8$ teaspoon ground cloves
- ½ teaspoon salt

Directions:
1. Place all ingredients in a food processor and blend until a smooth consistency is achieved. Makes a delicious fruit and veggie dip and can be added to smoothies, on toast, on pancakes and waffles.

Nutrition:
- Fat: 9.5 g
- Cholesterol 0 mg
- Sodium 117 mg
- Carbohydrates: 4.1 g
- Fiber 2.4 g
- Protein: 4 g

Keto Strawberry Jam

Preparation Time: 25 minutes
Cooking Time: 5 minutes
Servings: 18
Ingredients:
- 1 cup fresh strawberries, chopped
- 1 tablespoon lemon juice
- 4 teaspoons xylitol
- 1 tablespoon water

Directions:
1. Add all ingredients to a small saucepan and place over medium heat. Stir to combine and cook for about 15 minutes. Stir occasionally.
2. After 15 minutes are up, mash up strawberries with a potato masher or fork.
3. Pour into a heat-safe container such as a mason jar.
4. Allow cooling then cover with a lid and refrigerate. Can be stored in the refrigerator for up to 3 days. Goes great with toast and sweet sandwiches.

Nutrition:
- Fat: 0 g
- Cholesterol 0 mg
- Sodium 0 mg
- Carbohydrates: 1 g
- Fiber 0.2 g
- Protein: 0.1 g

Spicy Avocado Mayonnaise

Preparation Time: 10 minutes

Cooking Time: 10 minutes
Servings: 8
Ingredients:

- 2 ripe avocados, pitted and peeled
- ¼ jalapeno pepper, minced
- 2 tablespoons lemon juice
- ½ teaspoon onion powder
- 2 tablespoons fresh cilantro, chopped
- Salt to taste

Directions:

1. Add all ingredients to a food processor and blender until a smooth creamy consistency is achieved.

The jalapeno peppers can be foregone if you prefer a cooler mayo. Can be enjoyed in sandwiches, on toast, as a topping, in veggie wraps and salads.

Nutrition:

- Fat: 9.8 g
- Cholesterol 0 mg
- Sodium 23 mg
- Carbohydrates: 4.6 g
- Fiber 3.4 g
- Protein: 1 g

Green Coconut Butter

Preparation Time: 10 minutes
Cooking Time: 10 minutes
Servings: 8
Ingredients:

- 2 cups unsweetened shredded coconut
- 2 teaspoons matcha powder
- 1 tablespoon coconut oil

Directions:

1. Add shredded coconut to a food processor and blend for 5 minutes or until a smooth but runny consistency is achieved.
2. Add matcha powder and olive oil. Blend for 1 more minute.
3. Can be stored in an airtight container at room temperature for up to 2 weeks. Makes a delicious fruit dip and can be added to smoothies, on pancakes and toast.

Nutrition:

- Fat: 5.2 g
- Cholesterol 0 mg
- Sodium 3 mg
- Carbohydrates: 1.7 g
- Fiber 1.2 g
- Protein: 0.7 g

Keto Vegan Raw Cashew Cheese Sauce

Preparation Time: 5 minutes
Cooking Time: 5 minutes
Servings: 6
Ingredients:

- 1 cup raw cashews, soaked in water for at least 3 hours before making the recipe
- 2 tablespoons olive oil
- 2 tablespoon nutritional yeast
- ¼ teaspoon garlic powder
- 2 tablespoons fresh lemon juice
- ½ cup water
- Salt to taste

Directions:

1. To prepare cashews before making the sauce, boil 2 cups of water turn off the heat and add cashews. This can be allowed to soak overnight. Rinse and strained cashews. Discard water.
2. Add all ingredients to a food processor and blend until a smooth consistency is achieved. Can be used to make pizzas, over roasted veggies, in lasagna, as a dip and more.

Nutrition:

- Fat: 15.5 g
- Sodium 34 mg
- Carbohydrates: 9.23 g
- Protein: 5.1 g

Homemade Hummus

Preparation Time: 15 minutes
Cooking Time: 0 minutes
Servings: 8
Ingredients:

- 30 ounces (2 cans) garbanzo beans
- ⅓ cup chickpea liquid
- ½ cup tahini
- ¼ cup olive oil
- 2 lemons, juiced
- 2 teaspoons garlic, minced
- ½ teaspoon salt

Directions:

1. Add all ingredients to a blender.
2. Blend until smooth for about 30 seconds.
3. Transfer to an airtight container and sprinkle with additional seasonings or olive oil if desired.

Nutrition:

- Calories: 330
- Fat: 17 g
- Protein: 12 g
- Carbohydrates: 35 g

Pineapple Mint Salsa

Preparation Time: 10 minutes
Cooking Time: 0 minutes
Servings: 3
Ingredients:

- 1 pound (454 g) fresh pineapple, finely diced and juices reserved
- 1 bunch mint, leaves only, chopped
- 1 minced jalapeno, (optional)
- 1 white or red onion, finely diced
- Salt, to taste (optional)

Directions:

1. In a medium bowl, mix the pineapple with its juice, mint, jalapeno (if desired), and onion, and whisk well. Season with salt to taste, if desired.
2. Refrigerate in an airtight container for at least 2 hours to better mix the flavors.

Nutrition:

- Calories: 58
- Fat: 0.1 g
- Carbohydrates: 13.7 g
- Protein: 0.5 g
- Fiber 1.0 g

Chapter 10: Dessert & Sweet Treats

Cinnamon Apple Chips

Preparation Time: 10 minutes
Cooking Time: 8 minutes
Servings: 6
Ingredients:

- 3 granny smith apples, wash, core and thinly slice
- 1 teaspoon ground cinnamon
- A pinch salt

Directions:

1. Rub apple slices with cinnamon and salt then place them into the Air Fryer basket.
2. Cook at 390°Fahrenheit for 8 minutes. Turn halfway through.
3. Serve and enjoy.

Nutrition:

- Calories: 170 Protein: 4 g
- Fat: 1 g Carbohydrates: 6 g

Apple Chips with Dip

Preparation Time: 10 minutes
Cooking Time: 12 minutes
Servings: 4
Ingredients:

- 1 apple, thinly slice using a mandolin slicer
- 1 tablespoon almond butter
- ¼ cup plain yogurt
- 2 teaspoons olive oil
- 1 teaspoon ground cinnamon
- 1- 2 Drops liquid stevia

Directions:

1. Add apple slices, oil, and cinnamon to a large bowl and toss well.
2. Spray Air Fryer basket with cooking spray.
3. Place apple slices in an Air Fryer basket and cook at 375°Fahrenheit for 12 minutes. Turn after every 4 minutes.
4. Meanwhile, in a small bowl, mix together almond butter, yogurt, and sweetener.
5. Serve apple chips with dip and enjoy.

Nutrition:

- Calories: 253 Carbohydrates: 15 g
- Carbohydrates: 13 g Protein: 27 g
- Fat: 9 g Sugar 4 g
- Fiber 2 g

Delicious Spiced Apples

Preparation Time: 10 minutes
Cooking Time: 10 minutes
Servings: 6
Ingredients:

- 5-6 Small apples, sliced
- 1 teaspoon apple pie spice
- ½ cup erythritol
- 2 tablespoons coconut oil, melted

Directions:

1. Add apple slices in a mixing bowl and sprinkle sweetener, apple pie spice, and coconut oil over the apple and toss to coat.
2. Transfer apple slices in an Air Fryer dish. Place dish in Air Fryer basket and cook at 350°Fahrenheitfor 10 minutes.
3. Serve and enjoy.

Nutrition:

- Calories: 234
- Fat: 13.8 g
- Carbohydrates: 5.9 g
- Protein: 20 g

Tasty Cheese Bites

Preparation Time: 10 minutes
Cooking Time: 2 minutes
Servings: 16
Ingredients:

- 8 ounces cream cheese, softened
- 2 tablespoons erythritol
- ½ cup almond flour
- ½ teaspoon vanilla
- 4 tablespoons heavy cream
- ½ cup erythritol

Directions:

1. Add cream cheese, vanilla, ½ cup erythritol, and 2 tablespoons heavy cream in a stand mixer and mix until smooth.
2. Scoop cream cheese mixture onto the parchment-lined plate and place in the refrigerator for 1 hour.
3. In a small bowl, mix together almond flour and 2 tablespoons erythritol.
4. Dip cheesecake bites in remaining heavy cream and coat with almond flour mixture.
5. Place the cheesecake bites in the basket of the Air Fryer and fry for 2 minutes at 350°Fahrenheit.
6. Make sure cheesecake bites are frozen before air fry otherwise they will melt.
7. Drizzle with chocolate syrup and serve.

Nutrition:

- Calories: 383
- Fat: 19.8 g
- Carbohydrates: 28 g
- Protein: 23 g

Apple Chips

Preparation Time: 10 minutes
Cooking Time: 20 minutes
Servings: 2
Ingredients:

- 1 apple, sliced thinly
- Salt to taste
- ¼ teaspoon ground cinnamon

Directions:

1. Preheat the Air Fryer to 350°Fahrenheit.
2. Toss the apple slices in salt and cinnamon.
3. Add to the Air Fryer.
4. Let cool before serving.

Nutrition:

- Calories: 59
- Protein: 0.3 g
- Fat: 0.2 g
- Carbohydrates: 15.6 g

Gooey Cinnamon S'mores

Preparation Time: 5 minutes
Cooking Time: 3 minutes
Makes: 12 s'mores
Ingredients:

- 12 whole cinnamon graham crackers, halved
- 2 (1-½ ounces) chocolate bars, cut into 12 pieces
- 12 marshmallows

Directions:

1. Arrange 12 graham cracker squares in the air fry basket in a single layer.
2. Top each square with a piece of chocolate.
3. Place the basket on the bake position.
4. Select bake set the temperature to 350°Fahrenheit (180°Celsius) and the time to 3 minutes.
5. After 2 minutes, remove the basket and place a marshmallow on each piece of melted chocolate. Return the basket to the Air Fryer grill and continue to cook for another 1 minute.
6. Remove from the Air Fryer grill to a serving plate.
7. Serve topped with the remaining graham cracker squares

Nutrition:

- Calories: 234
- Fat: 13.8 g
- Carbohydrates: 5.9 g
- Protein: 20 g

Sweetened Plantains

Preparation Time: 5 minutes
Cooking Time: 8 minutes
Servings: 4
Ingredients:

- 2 ripe plantains, sliced
- 2 teaspoons avocado oil
- Salt to taste
- Maple syrup

Directions:

1. Toss the plantains in oil.
2. Season with salt.
3. Cook in the Air Fryer basket at 400°Fahrenheit for 10 minutes, shaking after 5 minutes. Drizzle with maple syrup before serving.

Nutrition:

- Calories: 125
- Protein: 1.2 g
- Fat: 0.6 g
- Carbohydrates: 32 g

Pear Crisp

Preparation Time: 10 minutes
Cooking Time: 25 minutes
Servings: 2
Ingredients:

- 1 cup flour
- 1 stick vegan butter
- 1 tablespoon cinnamon
- ½ cup sugar
- 2 pears, cubed

Directions:

1. Mix flour and butter to form a crumbly texture.
2. Add cinnamon and sugar.
3. Put the pears in the Air Fryer.
4. Pour and spread the mixture on top of the pears.
5. Cook at 350°Fahrenheit for 25 minutes.
6. Serve

Nutrition:

- Calories: 544
- Protein: 7.4 g
- Fat: 0.9 g
- Carbohydrates: 132.3 g

Easy Pears Dessert

Preparation Time: 10 minutes
Cooking Time: 25 minutes
Servings: 12
Ingredients:

- 6 big pears, cored and chopped
- ½ cup raisins
- 1 teaspoon ginger powder
- ¼ cup coconut sugar
- 1 teaspoon lemon zest, grated

Directions:

1. In a container that fits your Air Fryer, mix pears with raisins, ginger, sugar and lemon zest. Stir, introduce in the fryer and cook at 350°Fahrenheit for 25 minutes.
2. Divide into bowls and serve cold.
3. Enjoy!

Nutrition:

- Calories: 200
- Protein: 6 g
- Fat: 3 g
- Carbohydrates: 6 g

Vanilla Strawberry Mix

Preparation Time: 10 minutes
Cooking Time: 20 minutes
Servings: 10
Ingredients:

- 2 tablespoons lemon juice
- 2 pounds strawberries
- 4 cups coconut sugar
- 1 teaspoon cinnamon powder
- 1 teaspoon vanilla extract

Directions:

1. In a pot that fits your Air Fryer, mix strawberries with coconut sugar, lemon juice, cinnamon and vanilla, stir gently, introduce in the fryer and cook at 350°Fahrenheit for 20 minutes.
2. Divide into bowls and serve cold.
3. Enjoy!

Nutrition:

- Calories: 140
- Protein: 2 g
- Fat: 0 g
- Carbohydrates: 5 g

Sweet Bananas and Sauce

Preparation Time: 10 minutes
Cooking Time: 20 minutes
Servings: 4

Ingredients:

- ½ lemon juice
- 3 tablespoons agave nectar
- 1 tablespoon coconut oil
- 4 bananas, peeled and sliced diagonally
- ½ teaspoon cardamom seeds

Directions:

1. Arrange bananas in a pan that fits your Air Fryer, add agave nectar, lemon juice, oil and cardamom. Introduce in the fryer and cook at 360°Fahrenheit for 20 minutes.
2. Divide bananas and sauce between plates and serve.
3. Enjoy!

Nutrition:

- Calories: 210
- Protein: 3 g
- Fat: 1 g
- Carbohydrates: 8 g

Cinnamon Apples and Mandarin Sauce

Preparation Time: 10 minutes
Cooking Time: 20 minutes
Servings: 4
Ingredients:

- 4 apples, cored, peeled and cored
- 2 cups mandarin juice
- ¼ cup maple syrup
- 2 teaspoons cinnamon powder
- 1 tablespoon ginger, grated

Directions:

1. In a pot that fits your Air Fryer, mix apples with mandarin juice, maple syrup, cinnamon and ginger. Introduce them in the fryer and cook at 365°Fahrenheit for 20 minutes.
2. Divide apples mix between plates and serve warm.
3. Enjoy!

Nutrition:

- Calories: 170
- Protein: 4 g
- Fat: 1 g
- Carbohydrates: 6 g

Cocoa Berries Cream

Preparation Time: 10 minutes
Cooking Time: 10 minutes
Servings: 4
Ingredients:

- 3 tablespoons cocoa powder
- 14 ounces coconut cream

- 1 cup blackberries
- 1 cup raspberries
- 2 tablespoons stevia

Directions:
1. In a bowl, whisk cocoa powder with stevia and cream and stir.
2. Add raspberries and blackberries, toss gently, transfer to a pan that fits your Air Fryer. Introduce in the fryer and cook at 350°Fahrenheit for 10 minutes.
3. Divide into bowls and serve cold.
4. Enjoy!

Nutrition:
- Calories: 205
- Protein: 2 g
- Fat: 34 g
- Carbohydrates: 6 g

Sweet Vanilla Rhubarb

Preparation Time: 10 minutes
Cooking Time: 10 minutes
Servings: 4
Ingredients:
- 5 cups rhubarb, chopped
- 2 tablespoons coconut butter, melted
- $^1/_3$ cup water
- 1 tablespoon stevia
- 1 teaspoon vanilla extract

Directions:
1. Put rhubarb, ghee, water, stevia, and vanilla extract in a pan that fits your Air Fryer, introduce in the fryer and cook at 365°Fahrenheit for 10 minutes.
2. Divide into small bowls and serve cold.
3. Enjoy!

Nutrition:
- Calories: 103
- Protein: 2 g
- Fat: 2 g
- Carbohydrates: 6 g

Cherries and Rhubarb Bowls

Preparation Time: 10 minutes
Cooking Time: 35 minutes
Servings: 4
Ingredients:
- 2 cups cherries, pitted and halved
- 1 cup rhubarb, sliced
- 1 cup apple juice
- 2 tablespoons sugar
- ½ cup raisins

Directions:

1. In a pot that fits your Air Fryer, combine the cherries with the rhubarb and the other ingredients. Toss, cook at 330°Fahrenheit for 35 minutes. Divide into bowls; cool down, and serve.

Nutrition:
- Calories: 212 Protein: 7 g
- Fat: 8 g Carbohydrates: 13 g

Pumpkin Bowls

Preparation Time: 10 minutes
Cooking Time: 15 minutes
Servings: 4
Ingredients:
- 2 cups pumpkin flesh, cubed
- 1 cup heavy cream
- 1 teaspoon cinnamon powder
- 3 tablespoons sugar
- 1 teaspoon nutmeg, ground

Directions:
1. In a pot that fits your Air Fryer, combine the pumpkin with the cream and the other ingredients. Introduce it in the fryer and cook at 360°Fahrenheit for 15 minutes.
2. Divide into bowls and serve.

Nutrition:
- Calories: 212
- Protein: 7 g
- Fat: 5 g
- Carbohydrates: 15 g

Buttery Fennel and Garlic

Preparation Time: 10 minutes
Cooking Time: 5 minutes
Servings: 4
Ingredients:
- ½ stick butter
- 2 garlic cloves, sliced
- ½ teaspoon salt
- 1-½ pounds fennel bulbs, cut into wedges
- ¼ teaspoon ground black pepper
- ½ teaspoon cayenne
- ¼ teaspoon dried dill weed
- $^1/_3$ cup dry white wine
- $^2/_3$ cup stock

Directions:
1. Set your Power XL Deluxe to Saute mode and add butter, let it heat up.
2. Add garlic and cook for 30 seconds.
3. Add the rest of the ingredients.
4. Lock lid and cook on low pressure for 3 minutes.
5. Remove lid and serve.

6. Enjoy!

Nutrition:
- Calories: 111
- Fat: 6 g
- Saturated fat 2 g
- Carbohydrates: 2 g
- Fiber 2 g
- Sodium 317 mg
- Protein: 2 g

Glazed Banana

Preparation Time: 10 minutes
Cooking Time: 10 minutes
Servings: 4
Ingredients:
- 2 ripe bananas, peeled and sliced lengthwise
- 1 teaspoon fresh lime juice
- 4 teaspoons maple syrup
- $1/8$ teaspoon ground cinnamon

Directions:
1. Coat each banana half with lime juice.
2. Arrange the banana halves onto the greased "Baking pan" cut sides up.
3. Drizzle the banana halves with maple syrup and sprinkle with cinnamon.
4. Select "Air Fry" of Kalorik Maxx Air Fryer Oven and then adjust the temperature to 350°Fahrenheit.
5. Set the timer for 10 minutes and press "Start/Stop" to begin cooking.
6. When the unit beeps to show that it is preheated, insert the baking pan in the Kalorik oven.
7. When cooking time is complete, remove the baking pan from the Kalorik oven and serve immediately.

Nutrition:
- Calories: 70
- Fat: 0.2 g
- Saturated fat 0.1 g
- Cholesterol 0 mg
- Sodium 1 mg
- Carbohydrates: 18 g
- Fiber 1.6 g
- Sugar 11.2 g
- Protein: 0.6 g

Cranberry Cupcakes

Preparation Time: 15 minutes
Cooking Time: 15 minutes
Servings: 10

Ingredients:
- 4-½ ounces self-rising flour
- ½ teaspoon baking powder
- A pinch salt
- ½ ounce cream cheese, softened
- 4-¾ ounces butter, softened
- 4-¼ ounces caster sugar
- 2 eggs
- 2 teaspoons fresh lemon juice
- ½ cup fresh cranberries

Directions:
1. In a bowl, mix together the flour, baking powder, and salt.
2. In another bowl, mix together the cream cheese, and butter.
3. Add the sugar and beat until fluffy and light.
4. Add the eggs, one at a time, and whisk until just combined.
5. Add the flour mixture and stir until well combined.
6. Stir in the lemon juice.
7. Place the mixture into silicone cups and top each with cranberries evenly, pressing slightly.
8. Select "Air Fry" of Kalorik Maxx Air Fryer Oven and then adjust the temperature to 365°Fahrenheit.
9. Set the timer for 15 minutes and press "Start/Stop" to begin cooking.
10. When the unit beeps to show that it is preheated, place the cups over the airing rack and insert them in the Kalorik oven.
11. When cooking time is complete, remove the cups from the Kalorik oven and place them onto a wire rack to cool for about 10 minutes.
12. Carefully, invert the cupcakes onto the wire rack to completely cool before serving.

Nutrition:
- Calories: 209 Fat: 12.4 g
- Saturated fat 7.5 g Cholesterol 63 mg
- Sodium 110 mg Carbohydrates: 22.6 g
- Fiber 0.6 g Sugar 12.4 g Protein: 2.7 g

Zucchini Mug Cake

Preparation Time: 10 minutes
Cooking Time: 20 minutes
Servings: 1
Ingredients:
- ¼ cup whole-wheat pastry flour
- 1 tablespoon sugar
- ¼ teaspoon baking powder
- ¼ teaspoon ground cinnamon
- A pinch salt

- 2 teaspoons milk
- 2 tablespoons zucchini, grated and squeezed
- 2 tablespoons almonds, chopped
- 1 tablespoon raisins
- 2 teaspoons maple syrup

Directions:

1. In a bowl, mix together the flour, sugar, baking powder, cinnamon and salt.
2. Add the remaining ingredients and mix until well combined.
3. Place the mixture into a lightly greased ramekin.
4. Select "Bake" of Kalorik Maxx Air Fryer Oven and then adjust the temperature to 350°Fahrenheit.
5. Set the timer for 20 minutes and press "Start/Stop" to begin cooking.
6. When the unit beeps to show that it is preheated, place the ramekin over the airing rack and insert it in the Kalorik oven.
7. When cooking time is complete, remove the ramekin from the Kalorik oven and place it onto a wire rack to cool slightly before serving.

Nutrition:

- Calories: 310
- Fat: 7 g
- Saturated fat 0.9 g
- Cholesterol 3 mg
- Sodium 175 mg
- Carbohydrates: 57.5 g
- Fiber 3.2 g
- Sugar 27.5 g
- Protein: 7.2 g

Chocolate Brownies

Preparation Time: 15 minutes
Cooking Time: 15 minutes
Servings: 4
Ingredients:

- ½ cup all-purpose flour
- ¾ cup sugar
- 6 tablespoons cacao powder
- ¼ teaspoon baking powder
- ¼ teaspoon salt
- ¼ cup butter, melted
- 2 large eggs
- 1 tablespoon olive oil
- ½ teaspoon pure vanilla extract

Directions:

1. Grease a 7-inch baking dish generously. Set aside.
2. In a bowl, add all the ingredients and mix until well combined.

3. Place the mixture into the baking dish and with the back of a spoon, smooth the top surface.
4. Arrange the baking pan of the oven in the bottom of the Kalorik Digital Air Fryer Oven.
5. Select "Air Fry" of Kalorik Maxx Air Fryer Oven and then adjust the temperature to 320°Fahrenheit.
6. Set the timer for 30 minutes and press "Start/Stop" to begin cooking.
7. When the unit beeps to show it is preheated, place the baking dish over the baking pan and insert it in the Kalorik oven.
8. When cooking time is complete, remove the pan from the Kalorik oven and place it onto a wire rack to cool completely before cutting.
9. Cut the brownie into desired-sized squares and serve.

Nutrition:

- Calories: 367
- Fat: 19.2 g
- Saturated fat 9.5 g
- Cholesterol 124 mg
- Sodium 265 mg
- Carbohydrates: 53.6 g
- Fiber 2.7 g
- Sugar 37.8 g
- Protein: 6.4 g

Banana and Walnut Cake

Preparation Time: 10 minutes
Cooking Time: 25 minutes
Servings: 6
Ingredients:

- 1 pound (454 g) bananas, mashed
- 8 ounces (227 g) flour
- 6 ounces (170 g) sugar
- $^7/_2$ ounces (99 g) walnuts, chopped
- $^7/_2$ ounces (71 g) butter, melted

- 2 eggs, lightly beaten
- ¼ teaspoon baking soda

Directions:

1. Select the Bake function and preheat Maxx to 355°Fahrenheit (179°Celsius).
2. In a bowl, combine the sugar, butter, egg, flour, and baking soda with a whisk. Stir in the bananas and walnuts.
3. Transfer the mixture to a greased baking dish. Put the dish in the Air Fryer oven and bake for 10 minutes.

4. Reduce the temperature to 330°Fahrenheit (166°Celsius) and bake for another 15 minutes. Serve hot.

Nutrition:
- Calories: 70
- Fat: 0.2 g
- Saturated fat 0.1 g
- Cholesterol 0 mg
- Sodium 1 mg
- Carbohydrates: 18 g
- Fiber 1.6 g
- Sugar 11.2 g
- Protein: 0.6 g

Perfect Cinnamon Toast

Preparation Time: 10 minutes
Cooking Time: 5 minutes
Servings: 6
Ingredients:
- 2 teaspoons pepper
- 1-½ teaspoons vanilla extract
- 1-½ teaspoons cinnamon
- ½ cup sweetener choice
- 1 cup coconut oil
- 12 slices whole-wheat bread

Directions:
1. Melt coconut oil and mix with sweetener until dissolved. Mix in remaining ingredients minus bread till incorporated.
2. Spread mixture onto bread, covering all area.
3. Pour the coated pieces of bread into the oven rack/basket. Place the rack on the middle shelf of the Air fryer oven. Set temperature to 400°Fahrenheit, and set Time to 5 minutes.
4. Remove and cut diagonally.
5. Enjoy!

Nutrition:
- Calories: 124
- Fat: 2 g
- Protein: 0 g
- Sugar 4 g

Apple Pie in Air Fryer

Preparation Time: 5 minutes
Cooking Time: 35 minutes
Servings: 4
Ingredients:
- ½ teaspoon vanilla extract
- 1 beaten egg
- 1 large apple, chopped
- 1 Pillsbury refrigerator pie crust

- 1 tablespoon butter
- 1 tablespoon ground cinnamon
- 1 tablespoon raw sugar
- 2 tablespoons sugar
- 2 teaspoons lemon juice
- Baking spray

Directions:
1. Lightly grease baking pan of Air Fryer oven with cooking spray. Spread pie crust on the bottom of the pan up to the sides.
2. In a bowl, mix vanilla, sugar, cinnamon, lemon juice, and apples. Pour on top of pie crust. Top apples with butter slices.
3. Cover apples with the other pie crust. Pierce with the knife the tops of pie.
4. Spread beaten egg on top of crust and sprinkle sugar.
5. Cover with foil.
6. For 25 minutes, cook at 390°Fahrenheit.
7. Remove foil cook for 10 minutes at 330°Fahrenheit until tops are browned.
8. Serve and enjoy.

Nutrition:
- Calories: 372 Fat: 19 g
- Protein: 4.2 g
- Sugar 5 g

Banana Brownies

Preparation Time: 5 minutes
Cooking Time: 30 minutes
Servings: 12
Ingredients:
- 2 cups almond flour
- 2 teaspoons baking powder
- ½ teaspoon baking powder
- ½ teaspoon baking soda
- ½ teaspoon salt
- 1 over-ripe banana
- 3 large eggs
- ½ teaspoon stevia powder
- ¼ cup coconut oil
- 1 tablespoon vinegar
- ⅓ cup almond flour
- ⅓ cup cocoa powder

Directions:
1. Preheat the Air Fryer oven for 5 minutes.
2. Combine all ingredients in a food processor and pulse until well-combined.
3. Pour into a baking dish that will fit in the Air Fryer.

4. Place in the Air Fryer basket and cook for 30 minutes at 350°Fahrenheit or if a toothpick inserted in the middle comes out clean.

Nutrition:
- Calories: 75
- Fat: 6.5 g
- Protein: 1.7 g
- Sugar 2 g

Chocolate Souffle for Two

Preparation Time: 5 minutes
Cooking Time: 14 minutes
Servings: 2
Ingredients:
- 2 tablespoons almond flour
- ½ teaspoon vanilla
- 3 tablespoons sweetener
- 2 separated eggs
- ¼ cup melted coconut oil
- 3 ounces semi-sweet chocolate, chopped

Directions:
1. Brush coconut oil and sweetener onto ramekins.
2. Melt coconut oil and chocolate together.
3. Beat egg yolks well, adding vanilla and sweetener. Stir in flour and ensure there are no lumps.
4. Preheat the Air Fryer oven to 330°Fahrenheit.
5. Whisk egg whites till they reach peak state and fold them into chocolate mixture.
6. Pour batter into ramekins and place into the Air Fryer oven.
7. Cook 14 minutes.
8. Serve with powdered sugar dusted on top.

Nutrition:
- Calories: 238
- Fat: 6 g
- Protein: 1 g
- Sugar 4 g

Blueberry Lemon Muffins

Preparation Time: 5 minutes
Cooking Time: 10 minutes
Servings: 12
Ingredients:
- 1 teaspoon vanilla
- 1 lemon juice and zest
- 2 eggs
- 1 cup blueberries
- ½ cup cream
- ¼ cup avocado oil
- ½ cup monk fruit
- 2-½ cups almond flour

Directions:
1. Mix monk fruit and flour together.
2. In another bowl, mix vanilla, egg, lemon juice, and cream together. Add mixtures together and blend well.
3. Spoon batter into cupcake holders.
4. Place in Air Fryer oven. Bake 10 minutes at 320°Fahrenheit, checking at 6 minutes to ensure you don't overbake them.

Nutrition:
- Calories: 317
- Fat: 11 g
- Protein: 3 g
- Sugar 5 g

Baked Apple

Preparation Time: 5 minutes
Cooking Time: 20 minutes
Servings: 4
Ingredients:
- ¼ cup water
- ¼ teaspoon nutmeg
- ¼ teaspoon cinnamon
- 1-½ teaspoons melted ghee
- 2 tablespoons raisins
- 2 tablespoons chopped walnuts
- 1 medium apple

Directions:
1. Preheat your Air Fryer to 350°Fahrenheit.
2. Slice an apple in half and discard some of the flesh from the center.
3. Place into the frying pan.
4. Mix remaining ingredients together except water. Spoon mixture to the middle of apple halves.
5. Pour water overfilled apples.
6. Air Frying. Place pan with apple halves into the Kalorik Maxx Air Fryer, bake 20 minutes.

Nutrition:
- Calories: 199
- Fat: 9 g
- Protein: 1 g
- Sugar 3 g

Cinnamon Fried Bananas

Preparation Time: 5 minutes
Cooking Time: 10 minutes
Servings: 2-3
Ingredients:
- 1 cup panko breadcrumbs
- 3 tablespoon cinnamon
- ½ cup almond flour

- 3 egg whites
- 8 ripe bananas
- 3 tablespoon vegan coconut oil

Directions:
1. Heat coconut oil and add breadcrumbs. Mix around 2-3 minutes until golden. Pour into a bowl.
2. Peel and cut bananas in half. Roll half of each banana into flour, eggs, and crumb mixture.
3. Air Frying. Place into the Kalorik Maxx Air Fryer. Cook 10 minutes at 280°Fahrenheit.
4. A great addition to a healthy banana split!

Nutrition:
- Calories: 219
- Fat: 10 g
- Protein: 3 g
- Sugar 5 g

Awesome Chinese Doughnuts

Preparation Time: 10 minutes
Cooking Time: 8 minutes
Servings: 8
Ingredients:
- 1 tablespoon baking powder
- 1 tablespoon coconut oil
- ¾ cup coconut milk
- 6 teaspoons sugar
- 2 cup all-purpose flour
- ½ teaspoon sea salt

Directions:
1. Preheat the Air Fryer to 350°Fahrenheit.
2. Mix baking powder, flour, sugar, and salt in a bowl.
3. Add coconut oil and mix well. Add coconut milk and mix until well combined.
4. Knead the dough for 3-4 minutes.
5. Roll dough half-inch thick and using a cookie cutter cut doughnuts.
6. Place doughnuts in a cake pan and brush with oil. Place cake pan in Air Fryer basket and air fry doughnuts for 5 minutes. Turn doughnuts to the other side and air fry for 3 minutes more.
7. Serve and enjoy.

Nutrition:
- Calories: 259
- Fat: 15.9 g
- Carbohydrates: 27 g
- Protein: 3.8 g

Crispy Bananas

Preparation Time: 10 minutes
Cooking Time: 10 minutes

Servings: 4
Ingredients:
- 4 sliced ripe bananas
- 1 egg
- ½ cup breadcrumbs
- 1-½ tablespoons cinnamon sugar
- 1 tablespoon almond meal
- 1-½ tablespoons coconut oil
- 1 tablespoon crushed cashew
- ¼ cup cornflour

Directions:
1. Set the pan on fire to heat the coconut oil over medium heat and add breadcrumbs in the pan and stir for 3-4 minutes.
2. Remove pan from heat and transfer breadcrumbs to a bowl.
3. Add almond meal and crush cashew in breadcrumbs and mix well.
4. Dip banana half in cornflour then in egg and finally coat with breadcrumbs.
5. Place coated banana in Air Fryer basket. Sprinkle with cinnamon sugar.
6. Air fry at 350°Fahrenheit/176°Celsius for 10 minutes.
7. Serve and enjoy.

Nutrition:
- Calories: 282 Fat: 9 g
- Carbohydrates: 46 g
- Protein: 5 g

Air Fried Banana and Walnuts Muffins

Preparation Time: 10 minutes
Cooking Time: 10 minutes
Servings: 2
Ingredients:
- ¼ cup flour
- ½ teaspoon baking powder
- ¼ cup mashed banana
- ¼ cup butter
- 1 tablespoon chopped walnuts
- ¼ cup oats

Directions:
1. Spray four muffin molds with cooking spray and set them aside.
2. In a bowl, mix together mashed bananas, walnuts, sugar, and butter.
3. In another bowl, mix oat flour, and baking powder.
4. Combine the flour mixture with the banana mixture.
5. Pour batter into the muffin mold.

6. Place in Air Fryer basket and cook at 320°Fahrenheit/160°Celsius for 10 minutes.
7. Remove muffins from the Air Fryer and allow them to cool completely.
8. Serve and enjoy.

Nutrition:
- Calories: 192
- Fat: 12.3 g
- Carbohydrates: 19.4 g
- Protein: 1.9 g

Nutty Mix

Preparation Time: 5 minutes
Cooking Time: 4 minutes
Servings: 6
Ingredients:
- 2 cup mix nuts
- 1 teaspoon ground cumin
- 1 teaspoon chili powder
- 1 tablespoon melted butter
- 1 teaspoon salt
- 1 teaspoon pepper

Directions:
1. Set all ingredients in a large bowl and toss until well coated.
2. Preheat the Air Fryer at 350°Fahrenheit for 5 minutes.
3. Add mix nuts in the Air Fryer basket and air fry for 4 minutes. Shake basket halfway through.
4. Serve and enjoy.

Nutrition:
- Calories: 316
- Fat: 29 g
- Carbohydrates: 11.3 g
- Protein: 7.6 g

Chocolate Cup Cakes

Preparation Time: 5 minutes
Cooking Time: 12 minutes
Servings: 6
Ingredients:
- 3 eggs
- ¼ cup caster sugar
- ¼ cup cocoa powder
- 1 teaspoon baking powder
- 1 cup milk
- ¼ teaspoon vanilla essence
- 2 cup all-purpose flour
- 4 tablespoons butter

Directions:
1. Preheat your Air Fryer to a temperature of 400°Fahrenheit (200°Celsius).

2. Beat eggs with sugar in a bowl until creamy.
3. Add butter and beat again for 1-2 minutes.
4. Now add flour, cocoa powder, milk, baking powder, and vanilla essence, mix with a spatula.
5. Fill ¾ of muffin tins with the mixture and place them into the Air Fryer basket.
6. Let cook for 12 minutes.
7. Serve!

Nutrition:
- Calories: 289
- Fat: 11.5 g
- Carbohydrates: 38.94 g
- Protein: 8.72 g

Air Roasted Nuts

Preparation Time: 10 minutes
Cooking Time: 20 minutes
Servings: 8
Ingredients:
- 1 cup raw peanuts
- ½ teaspoon cayenne pepper
- 3 teaspoons seafood seasoning
- 2 tablespoons olive oil
- Salt to taste

Directions:
1. Preheat your Air Fryer toast oven to 320°Fahrenheit.
2. In a bowl, whisk together cayenne pepper, olive oil, and seafood seasoning; stir in peanuts until well coated.
3. Transfer to the fryer basket and air roast for 10 minutes; toss well and then cook for another 10 minutes.
4. Transfer the peanuts to a dish and season with salt. Let cool before serving.

Nutrition:
- Calories: 193
- Fat: 17.4 g
- Carbohydrates: 4.9 g
- Protein: 7.4 g

Air Fried White Corn

Preparation Time: 10 minutes
Cooking Time: 40 minutes
Servings: 8
Ingredients:
- 2 cups giant white corn
- 3 tablespoons olive oil
- 1-½ teaspoons sea salt

Directions:
1. Soak the corn in a bowl of water for at least 8 hours or overnight; drain and spread in a single layer on a baking tray; pat dry with paper towels.

2. Preheat your Air Fryer toast oven to 400°Fahrenheit.
3. In a bowl, mix corn, olive oil, and salt and toss to coat well.
4. Air fry corn in batches in the preheated Air Fryer toast oven for 20 minutes, shaking the basket halfway through cooking.

5. Let the corn cool for at least 20 minutes or until crisp.

Nutrition:
- Calories: 225
- Fat: 7.4 g
- Carbohydrates: 35.8 g
- Protein: 5.9 g

Chapter 11: Cakes, Pies, and Muffins

Sponge Cake

Preparation Time: 10 minutes
Cooking Time: 40 minutes
Servings: 12
Ingredients:

- 4 eggs
- ½ cup swerve
- 2 cups almond flour
- 1 teaspoon vanilla
- 1 cup margarine

Directions:

1. Preheat the Air Fryer to 350°Fahrenheit.
2. Grease Air Fryer cake pan with cooking spray and set aside.
3. In a large bowl, beat margarine and sweetener using a hand mixer until light and fluffy.
4. Add egg one by one and beat well.
5. Add vanilla and almond flour and mix until well combined.
6. Pour batter into the pan and place into the Air Fryer.
7. Cook for 40 minutes.
8. Slice and serve.

Nutrition:

- Calories: 140
- Protein: 2 g
- Fat: 0 g
- Carbohydrates: 5 g

Almond Coconut Lemon Cake

Preparation Time: 10 minutes
Cooking Time: 48 minutes
Servings: 10
Ingredients:

- 4 eggs
- 2 tablespoons lemon zest
- ½ cup butter softened
- 2 teaspoons baking powder
- ¼ cup coconut flour
- 2 cups almond flour
- ½ cup fresh lemon juice
- ¼ cup swerve
- 1 tablespoon vanilla

Directions:

1. Preheat the Air Fryer to 280°Fahrenheit.
2. Grease Air Fryer baking dish with cooking spray and set aside.
3. In a large bowl, beat all ingredients using a hand mixer until smooth.
4. Pour batter into the dish and place into the Air Fryer and cook for 48 minutes.
5. Slice and serve.

Nutrition:

- Calories: 212
- Protein: 7 g
- Fat: 8 g
- Carbohydrates: 13 g

Vanilla Butter Cheese Cake

Preparation Time: 10 minutes
Cooking Time: 32 minutes
Servings: 9
Ingredients:

- 5 eggs
- 1 cup erythritol
- 4 ounces cream cheese, softened
- 1 teaspoon vanilla
- 1 teaspoon baking powder
- 6-½ ounces almond flour
- ½ cup butter, softened

Directions:

1. Preheat the Air Fryer to 325°Fahrenheit.
2. Grease Air Fryer baking dish with cooking spray and set aside.
3. Add all ingredients into the large bowl and beat until fluffy.
4. Pour batter into the pan and place into the Air Fryer and cook for 32 minutes.
5. Slice and serve.

Nutrition:

- Calories: 367
- Protein: 2 g
- Fat: 7 g
- Carbohydrates: 10 g

Almond Cinnamon Mug Cake

Preparation Time: 5 minutes
Cooking Time: 10 minutes
Servings: 1
Ingredients:
- 1 scoop vanilla protein powder
- ½ teaspoon cinnamon
- 1 teaspoon granulated sweetener
- 1 tablespoon almond flour
- ½ teaspoon baking powder
- ¼ teaspoon vanilla
- ¼ cup unsweetened almond milk

Directions:
1. Add protein powder, cinnamon, almond flour, sweetener, and baking powder into the mug and mix well.
2. Add vanilla and almond milk and stir well.
3. Place the mug in the Air Fryer and cook at 390°Fahrenheit for 10 minutes.
4. Serve and enjoy.

Nutrition:
- Calories: 140
- Protein: 2 g
- Fat: 0 g
- Carbohydrates: 5 g

Chocolate Coconut Cake

Preparation Time: 10 minutes
Cooking Time: 20 minutes
Servings: 9
Ingredients:
- 6 eggs
- 2 teaspoons baking powder
- 3 ounces unsweetened cocoa powder
- 5 ounces erythritol
- 2 cups coconut flour
- 1 Teaspoon vanilla
- 1 cup butter, melted
- 11 ounces heavy cream

Directions:
1. Preheat the Air Fryer to 325°Fahrenheit.
2. In a bowl, mix together coconut flour, butter, 5 ounces heavy cream, eggs, baking powder half cocoa powder, and 3 ounces sweetener until well combined.
3. Pour batter into the greased cake pan and place into the Air Fryer.ook for 20 minutes.
4. Allow cooling completely.
5. In a large bowl, beat the remaining heavy cream, cocoa powder, and sweetener until smooth.

6. Spread the cream on top of the cake and place it in the refrigerator for 30 minutes.
7. Slice and serve.

Nutrition:
- Calories: 212
- Protein: 7 g
- Fat: 8 g
- Carbohydrates: 13 g

Choco Fudge Cake

Preparation Time: 10 minutes
Cooking Time: 24 minutes
Servings: 12
Ingredients:
- 6 eggs
- ½ cup swerve
- 1- Ounce unsweetened chocolate, melted
- ½ cup almond flour
- 11 Ounce butter, melted pinch salt

Directions:
1. Preheat the Air Fryer to 325°Fahrenheit.
2. Grease Air Fryer baking dish with cooking spray and set aside.
3. In a large bowl, beat eggs until foamy. Add sweetener and stir well.
4. Add melted butter, chocolate, almond flour, and salt and stir to combine.
5. Pour batter into the pan and place into the Air Fryer and cook for 24 minutes.
6. Slice and serve.

Nutrition:
- Calories: 367
- Protein: 2 g
- Fat: 7 g
- Carbohydrates: 10 g

Cranberry Almond Cake

Preparation Time: 10 minutes
Cooking Time: 16 minutes
Servings: 6
Ingredients:
- 4 eggs
- 1 teaspoon orange zest
- 2 teaspoons mixed spice
- 2 teaspoons cinnamon
- ¼ cup swerve
- 1 Cup butter, softened
- ⅔ cup dried cranberries
- 1-½ cups almond flour
- 1 teaspoon vanilla

Directions:
1. Preheat the Air Fryer to 325°Fahrenheit.

2. In a bowl, add sweetener and melted butter and beat until fluffy.
3. Add cinnamon, vanilla, and mixed spice and stir well.
4. Add eggs stir until well combined.
5. Add almond flour, orange zest, and cranberries and stir to combine.
6. Pour batter in a greased Air Fryer cake pan and place it into the Air Fryer.
7. Cook cake for 16 minutes.
8. Slice and serve.

Nutrition:
- Calories: 140
- Protein: 2 g
- Fat: 0 g
- Carbohydrates: 5 g

Pumpkin Custard

Preparation Time: 10 minutes
Cooking Time: 32 minutes
Servings: 6
Ingredients:
- 4 egg yolks
- ½ teaspoon cinnamon
- 15 drops liquid stevia
- 15 ounces pumpkin puree
- ¾ cup coconut cream
- ⅛ teaspoon cloves
- ⅛ teaspoon ginger

Directions:
1. Preheat the Air Fryer to 325°Fahrenheit.
2. In a large bowl, combine together pumpkin puree, cinnamon, swerve, cloves, and ginger.
3. Add egg yolks and beat until combined.
4. Add coconut cream and stir well.
5. Pour mixture into the six ramekins and place into the Air Fryer.
6. Cook for 32 minutes.
7. Let it cool completely then place it in the refrigerator.
8. Serve chilled and enjoy.

Nutrition:
- Calories: 170
- Protein: 4 g
- Fat: 1 g
- Carbohydrates: 6 g

Angel Food Cake

Preparation Time: 5 minutes
Cooking Time: 30 minutes
Servings: 12
Ingredients:

- ¼ cup butter, melted
- 1 cup powdered erythritol
- 1 teaspoon strawberry extract
- 12 egg whites
- 2 teaspoons cream tartar

Directions:
1. Preheat the Air Fryer oven for 5 minutes. Blend the cream of tartar and egg whites.
2. Use a hand mixer and whisk until white and fluffy.
3. Add the rest of the ingredients, except for the butter and whisk for another minute.
4. Pour into a baking dish.
5. Place in the Air Fryer basket and cook for 30 minutes at 400°Fahrenheit or until a toothpick inserted in the middle comes out clean.
6. Drizzle with melted butter once cooled.

Nutrition:
- Calories: 65
- Protein: 3.1 g
- Fat: 5 g
- Carbohydrates: 6.2 g

Strawberry Cheese Cake

Preparation Time: 10 minutes
Cooking Time: 35 minutes
Servings: 6
Ingredients:
- 1 cup almond flour
- 3 tablespoon coconut oil, melted
- ½ teaspoon vanilla
- 1 egg, lightly beaten
- 1 tablespoon fresh lime juice
- ¼ cup erythritol
- 1 cup cream cheese, softened
- 1 pound strawberries, chopped
- 2 teaspoon baking powder

Directions:
1. Add all ingredients into the large bowl and mix until well combined.
2. Grease Air Fryer baking dish with cooking spray.
3. Pour batter into the pan and place into the Air Fryer and cook at 350°Fahrenheitfor for 35 minutes.
4. Allow cooling completely.

Nutrition:
- Calories: 140
- Protein: 2 g
- Fat: 0 g

- Carbohydrates: 5 g

Easy Orange Coconut Cake

Preparation Time: 5 minutes
Cooking Time: 17 minutes
Servings: 6
Ingredients:

- 1 stick butter, melted
- ¾ cup granulated swerve
- 2 eggs, beaten
- ¾ cup coconut flour
- ¼ teaspoon salt
- ⅓ teaspoon grated nutmeg
- ⅓ cup coconut milk
- 1-¼ cups almond flour
- ½ teaspoon baking powder
- 2 tablespoons unsweetened orange jam
- Cooking spray

Directions:

1. Coat a baking pan with cooking spray. Set aside.
2. In a large mixing bowl, whisk together the melted butter and granulated swerve until fluffy.
3. Mix in the beaten eggs and whisk again until smooth. Stir in the salt, nutmeg, and coconut flour and gradually pour in the coconut milk. Add the remaining ingredients and stir until well incorporated.
4. Scrape the batter into the baking pan.
5. Place the pan on the bake position.
6. Select bake, set the temperature to 355°Fahrenheit (179°Celsius), and set time to 17 minutes.
7. When cooking is complete, the top of the cake should spring back when gently pressed with your fingers.
8. Remove from the Air Fryer grill to a wire rack to cool. Serve chilled.

Nutrition:

- Calories: 367 Protein: 2 g
- Fat: 7 g
- Carbohydrates: 10 g

Easy Lava Cake

Preparation Time: 10 minutes
Cooking Time: 9 minutes
Servings: 2
Ingredients:

- 1 egg
- ½ teaspoon baking powder
- 1 tablespoon coconut oil, melted

- 1 tablespoon flax meal
- 2 tablespoons erythritol
- 3-4 Tablespoon water
- 2 tablespoons unsweetened cocoa powder pinch salt

Directions:

1. Whisk all ingredients into the bowl and transfer in two ramekins.
2. Preheat the Air Fryer to 350°Fahrenheit.
3. Place ramekins in Air Fryer basket and bake for 8-9 minutes.
4. Carefully remove ramekins from the Air Fryer and let it cool for 10 minutes.
5. Serve and enjoy.

Nutrition:

- Calories: 65
- Protein: 3.1 g
- Fat: 5 g
- Carbohydrates: 6.2 g

Choco Mug Cake

Preparation Time: 5 minutes
Cooking Time: 20 minutes
Servings: 1
Ingredients:

- 1 egg, lightly beaten
- 1 tablespoon heavy cream
- ¼ teaspoon baking powder
- 2 tablespoons unsweetened cocoa powder
- 2 tablespoon erythritol
- ½ teaspoon vanilla
- 1 tablespoon peanut butter
- 1 teaspoon salt

Directions:

1. Preheat the Air Fryer to 400°Fahrenheit.
2. In a bowl, mix together all ingredients until well combined.
3. Spray mug with cooking spray.
4. Pour batter in mug and place in the Air Fryer and cook for 20 minutes.
5. Serve and enjoy.

Nutrition:

- Calories: 212 Protein: 7 g
- Fat: 8 g Carbohydrates: 13 g

Chocolate Custard

Preparation Time: 10 minutes
Cooking Time: 32 minutes
Servings: 4
Ingredients:

- 2 eggs
- 1 Teaspoon vanilla

- 1 cup heavy whipping cream
- 1 cup unsweetened almond milk
- 1 Tablespoon unsweetened cocoa powder
- ¼ cup swerves pinch salt

Directions:
1. Preheat the Air Fryer to 305°Fahrenheit.
2. Add all ingredients into the blender and blend until well combined.
3. Pour mixture into the ramekins and place into the Air Fryer.
4. Cook for 32 minutes.
5. Serve and enjoy.

Nutrition:
- Calories: 212 Protein: 7 g
- Fat: 8 g
- Carbohydrates: 13 g

Delicious Vanilla Custard

Preparation Time: 10 minutes
Cooking Time: 20 minutes
Servings: 2
Ingredients:
- 2 Eggs
- 2 tablespoons swerve
- 1 teaspoon vanilla
- ½ cup unsweetened almond milk
- ½ cup cream cheese

Directions:
1. Add eggs to a bowl and beat using a hand mixer.
2. Add cream cheese, sweetener, vanilla, and almond milk and beat for 2 minutes more.
3. Spray two ramekins with cooking spray.
4. Pour batter into the ramekins.
5. Preheat the Air Fryer to 350°Fahrenheit.
6. Place ramekins into the Air Fryer and cook for 20 minutes.
7. Serve and enjoy.

Nutrition:
- Calories: 212
- Protein: 7 g
- Fat: 8 g
- Carbohydrates: 13 g

Honey Graham Crackers Pie

Preparation Time: 10 minutes
Cooking Time: 45 minutes
Servings: 8
Ingredients:
- 2 cups self-rising flour
- 1 cup almond flour
- 1 teaspoon baking powder

- ½ cup butter, softened
- ½ cup packed brown sugar
- ⅓ cup honey
- 1 teaspoon vanilla extract
- ½ cup coconut milk

Directions:
1. Sieve self-rising flour, almond flour, baking powder, and baking powder; keep separately. In a medium container, stir gently and loosely butter, brown sugar and honey. Add the sifted ingredients alternately with milk and vanilla.
2. Cover the dough and cool it overnight. Preheat the Air Fryer toaster oven to 175°Celsius. Divide the cold dough into quarters.
3. Spread the dough on a well-floured surface quarterly in a 5x15 inch rectangle. Divide into rectangles with a knife. Place rectangles on non-greased baking sheets. Draw a line in the middle and click with a fork.
4. For a cinnamon biscuit, sprinkle with a mixture of sugar and cinnamon before baking. Bake in the preheated oven for 13 to 15 minutes. Remove the baking trays to cool them on racks.

Nutrition:
- Calories: 120
- Fat: 3.9 g
- Carbohydrates: 1.9 g
- Protein: 1.9 g

Peach Pie Mix

Preparation Time: 15 minutes
Cooking Time: 35 minutes
Servings: 5
Ingredients:
- 1 tablespoon dark rum
- 1 pie dough
- 2 tablespoons cornstarch
- 1 tsp Ground nutmeg
- 2 tablespoons butter
- 2 tablespoons flour
- 2-¼ pounds peaches
- 1 tablespoon lemon juice
- ½ cup sugar

Directions:
1. Press the dough on the Power XL Air Fryer Grill pan.
2. Mix sugar, nutmeg, lemon juice, cornstarch, and butter in a bowl.
3. Add peaches, rum, and flour.
4. Mix well.
5. Pour the mixture into the dough.

6. Set the Power XL Air Fryer Grill to toast/bagel function.
7. Cook for 35 minutes at 350°Fahrenheit.
8. Serve immediately or allow cooling before serving.

Serving suggestions: Serve with orange juice.

Directions and cooking tips: Mix ingredients well.

Nutrition:
- Calories: 261
- Fat: 12 g
- Carbohydrates: 39 g
- Proteins 3 g

Southern Fudge Pie

Preparation Time: 15 minutes
Cooking Time: 26 minutes
Servings: 8
Ingredients:
- 1-½ cups sugar
- ½ cup self-rising flour
- ⅓ cup unsweetened cocoa powder
- 3 large eggs, beaten
- 12 tablespoons (1-½ sticks) butter, melted
- 1-½ teaspoons vanilla extract
- 1 (9-inch) unbaked pie crust
- ¼ cup confectioners' sugar (optional)

Directions:
1. Thoroughly combine the flour, cocoa powder, and sugar in a medium bowl. Add the beaten eggs and butter and whisk to combine. Stir in the vanilla.
2. Pour the filling into the pie crust and transfer it to the air fry basket.
3. Place the basket on the bake position.
4. Select bake set the temperature to 350°Fahrenheit (180°Celsius) and set time to 26 minutes.
5. When cooking is complete, the pie should be set.
6. Allow the pie to cool for 5 minutes. Sprinkle with the confectioners' sugar, if desired. Serve warm.

Nutrition:
- Calories: 212
- Protein: 7 g
- Fat: 8 g
- Carbohydrates: 13 g

Cashew Pie

Preparation Time: 10 minutes
Cooking Time: 18 minutes
Servings: 8

Ingredients:
- 1 egg
- 2 ounces cashews, crushed
- ½ teaspoon baking soda
- ⅓ cup heavy cream
- 1-ounce dark chocolate, melted
- 1 tablespoon butter
- 1 teaspoon vinegar
- 1 cup coconut flour

Directions:
1. Add egg in a bowl and beat using a hand mixer. Add coconut flour and stir well.
2. Add butter, vinegar, baking soda, heavy cream, and melted chocolate. Stir well.
3. Add cashews and mix well.
4. Preheat the Air Fryer to 350°Fahrenheit.
5. Add dough to an Air Fryer baking dish and flatten it into a pie shape.
6. Cook for 18 minutes.
7. Slice and serve.

Nutrition:
- Calories: 212
- Protein: 7 g
- Fat: 8 g
- Carbohydrates: 13 g

Vanilla Butter Pie

Preparation Time: 10 minutes
Cooking Time: 20 minutes
Servings: 8
Ingredients:
- 1 egg
- 2 tablespoons erythritol
- ½ cup butter, melted
- 1 teaspoon vanilla
- 1 cup almond flour
- 1 teaspoon baking soda
- 1 tablespoon vinegar

Directions:
1. Mix together almond flour and baking soda in a bowl.
2. In a separate bowl, whisk the egg with sweetener and vanilla.
3. Pour whisk egg, vinegar, and butter in almond flour and mix until dough is formed.
4. Preheat the Air Fryer to 340°Fahrenheit.
5. Roll dough using the rolling pin in Air Fryer baking dish size.
6. Place rolled dough in an Air Fryer baking dish. Place in the Air Fryer and cook for 20 minutes.
7. Slice and serve.

Nutrition:

- Calories: 140
- Protein: 2 g
- Fat: 0 g
- Carbohydrates: 5 g

Bourbon Chocolate Pecan Pie

Preparation Time: 20 minutes
Cooking Time: 25 minutes
Servings: 8
Ingredients:
- 1 (9-inch) unbaked pie crust

Filling:
- 2 large eggs
- $^{1}/_{3}$ cup butter, melted
- 1 cup sugar
- ½ cup all-purpose flour
- 1 cup milk chocolate chips
- 1-½ cups coarsely chopped pecans
- 2 tablespoons bourbon

Directions:
1. Whisk the eggs and melted butter in a large bowl until creamy.
2. Add the flour and sugar and stir to combine. Mix in the pecans, milk chocolate chips, and bourbon and stir until well blended.
3. Use a fork to prick holes in the bottom and sides of the pie crust. Pour the filling into the pie crust. Place the pie crust in the air fry basket.
4. Place the basket on the bake position.
5. Select bake set the temperature to 350°Fahrenheit (180°Celsius) and set Time to 25 minutes.
6. When cooking is complete, a toothpick inserted in the center should come out clean.
7. Allow the pie to cool for 10 minutes in the basket before serving.

Nutrition:
- Calories: 140
- Protein: 2 g
- Fat: 0 g
- Carbohydrates: 5 g

Chocolate Pudding

Preparation Time: 10 minutes
Cooking Time: 10 minutes
Servings: 8
Ingredients:
- 1 egg
- 1 egg yolk
- ¾ cup chocolate milk
- 3 tablespoons brown sugar

- 3 tablespoons peanut butter
- 2 tablespoons cocoa powder
- 1 teaspoon vanilla
- 5 slices firm white bread, cubed
- Non-stick cooking spray

Directions:
1. Spritz a baking pan with non-stick cooking spray.
2. Whisk together the egg yolk, egg, peanut butter, chocolate milk, cocoa powder, brown sugar, and vanilla until well combined.
3. Fold in the bread cubes and stir to mix well. Allow the bread to soak for 10 minutes.
4. When ready, transfer the egg mixture to the baking pan.
5. Place the pan on the bake position.
6. Select bake set the temperature to 330°Fahrenheit (166°Celsius) and set the time to 10 minutes.
7. When done, the pudding should be just firm to the touch.
8. Serve at room temperature.

Nutrition:
- Calories: 367
- Protein: 2 g
- Fat: 7 g
- Carbohydrates: 10 g

Coconut Pie

Preparation Time: 10 minutes
Cooking Time: 12 minutes
Servings: 6
Ingredients:
- 2 eggs
- ½ cup coconut flour
- ½ cup erythritol
- 1 cup shredded coconut
- 1-½ teaspoon vanilla
- ¼ cup butter
- 1-½ cups coconut milk

Directions:
1. Add all ingredients into the large bowl and mix until well combined.
2. Spray a 6-inch baking dish with cooking spray.
3. Pour batter into the dish and place in the Air Fryer basket.
4. Cook at 350°Fahrenheitfor 10-12 minutes.
5. Slice and serve.

Nutrition:
- Calories: 212 Protein: 7 g
- Fat: 8 g Carbohydrates: 13 g

Pumpkin Muffins

Preparation Time: 10 minutes
Cooking Time: 20 minutes
Servings: 10
Ingredients:

- Large eggs
- ½ cup pumpkin puree
- 1 tablespoon pumpkin pie spice
- 1 tablespoon baking powder, gluten-free
- ⅔ cup erythritol
- 1 teaspoon vanilla
- ⅓ cup coconut oil, melted
- ½ cup almond flour
- ½ cup coconut flour
- ½ teaspoon sea salt

Directions:

1. Preheat the Air Fryer to 325°Fahrenheit.
2. In a large bowl, stir together coconut flour, pumpkin pie spice, baking powder, erythritol, almond flour, and sea salt.
3. Stir in eggs, vanilla, coconut oil, and pumpkin puree until well combined.
4. Pour batter into the silicone muffin molds and place it into the Air Fryer basket in batches.
5. Cook muffins for 20 minutes.

Nutrition:

- Calories: 278 Protein: 5 g
- Fat: 10 g
- Carbohydrates: 17 g

Cappuccino Muffins

Preparation Time: 10 minutes
Cooking Time: 20 minutes
Servings: 12
Ingredients:

- 4 eggs
- 2 cups almond flour
- ½ teaspoon vanilla
- 1 teaspoon espresso powder
- ½ cup sour cream
- 1 teaspoon cinnamon
- 2 teaspoons baking powder
- ¼ cup coconut flour
- ½ cup swerve
- ¼ teaspoon salt

Directions:

1. Preheat the Air Fryer to 325°Fahrenheit.
2. Add sour cream, vanilla, espresso powder, and eggs in a blender and blend until smooth.

3. Add almond flour, cinnamon, baking powder, coconut flour, sweetener, and salt. Blend again until smooth.
4. Pour batter into the silicone muffin molds and place it into the Air Fryer basket. (cook in batches)
5. Cook muffins for 20 minutes.
6. Serve

Nutrition:

- Calories: 367
- Protein: 2 g
- Fat: 7 g
- Carbohydrates: 10 g

Moist Cinnamon Muffins

Preparation Time: 10 minutes
Cooking Time: 12 minutes
Servings: 20
Ingredients:

- 1 tablespoon cinnamon
- 1 teaspoon baking powder
- 2 scoops vanilla protein powder
- ½ cup almond flour
- ½ cup coconut oil
- ½ cup pumpkin puree
- ½ cup almond butter

Directions:

1. Preheat the Air Fryer to 325°Fahrenheit.
2. In a large bowl, combine together all dry ingredients and mix well.
3. Add wet ingredients into the dry ingredients and mix until well combined.
4. Pour batter into the silicone muffin molds and place it into the Air Fryer basket (cook in batches).
5. Cook muffins for 12 minutes.
6. Serve

Nutrition:

- Calories: 212
- Protein: 7 g
- Fat: 8 g
- Carbohydrates: 13 g

Cream Cheese Muffins

Preparation Time: 10 minutes
Cooking Time: 16 minutes
Servings: 10
Ingredients:

- 2 eggs
- ½ cup erythritol
- 8 ounces cream cheese
- 1 teaspoon ground cinnamon

- ½ teaspoon vanilla

Directions:
1. Preheat the Air Fryer to 325°Fahrenheit.
2. In a bowl, mix together cream cheese, vanilla, erythritol, and eggs until soft.
3. Pour batter into the silicone muffin molds and sprinkle cinnamon on top.
4. Place muffin molds into the Air Fryer basket and cook for 16 minutes.

Nutrition:
- Calories: 140
- Protein: 2 g
- Fat: 0 g
- Carbohydrates: 5 g

Strawberry Muffins

Preparation Time: 10 minutes
Cooking Time: 15 minutes
Servings: 12
Ingredients:
- 3 eggs
- 1 teaspoon ground cinnamon
- 2 teaspoon baking powder
- 2-½ cups almond flour
- ⅔ cup fresh strawberries, diced
- ⅓ cup heavy cream
- 1 teaspoon vanilla
- ½ cup swerve
- 5 tablespoons butter

Directions:
1. Preheat the Air Fryer to 325°Fahrenheit.
2. Add butter and sweetener to a bowl and beat using a hand mixer until smooth.
3. Add eggs, cream, and vanilla and beat until frothy.
4. In another bowl, sift together almond flour, cinnamon, baking powder, and salt.
5. Add almond flour mixture to wet ingredients and mix until well combined.
6. Add strawberries and fold well.
7. Pour batter into the silicone muffin molds and place it into the Air Fryer basket in batches.
8. Cook muffins for 15 minutes.
9. Serve

Nutrition:
- Calories: 367
- Protein: 2 g
- Fat: 7 g
- Carbohydrates: 10 g

Pecan Muffins

Preparation Time: 10 minutes

Cooking Time: 15 minutes
Servings: 12
Ingredients:
- 4 eggs
- 1 teaspoon vanilla
- ¼ cup almond milk
- 2 tablespoons butter, melted
- ½ cup swerve
- 1 teaspoon psyllium husk
- 1 tablespoon baking powder
- ½ cup pecans, chopped
- ½ teaspoon ground cinnamon
- 2 teaspoons allspice
- 1-½ cups almond flour

Directions:
1. Preheat the Air Fryer to 370°Fahrenheit.
2. Beat eggs, almond milk, vanilla, sweetener, and butter in a bowl using a hand mixer until smooth.
3. Add remaining ingredients and mix until well combined.
4. Pour batter into the silicone muffin molds and place it into the Air Fryer basket in batches.
5. Cook muffins for 15 minutes.
6. Serve

Nutrition:
- Calories: 357 Protein: 3 g
- Fat: 8 g Carbohydrates: 12 g

Blackberry Muffins

Preparation Time: 5 minutes
Cooking Time: 12 minutes
Servings: 8
Ingredients:
- ½ cup fresh blackberries
- 1-½ cups almond flour
- 1 teaspoon baking powder
- ½ teaspoon baking soda
- ½ cup swerve
- ¼ teaspoon kosher salt
- 2 eggs
- ¼ cup coconut oil, melted
- ½ cup milk
- ½ teaspoon vanilla paste

Directions:
1. Line an 8 cups muffin tin with paper liners.
2. Thoroughly combine the almond flour, salt, swerve, baking powder, and baking soda in a mixing bowl.
3. Whisk together the eggs, milk, vanilla, and

coconut oil in a separate mixing bowl until smooth.

4. Add the wet mixture to the dry and fold in the blackberries. Stir with a spatula just until well incorporated.
5. Spoon the batter into the muffin cups, filling each about three-quarters full.
6. Place the muffin tin on the bake position.
7. Select bake set the temperature to 350°Fahrenheit (180°Celsius) and set Time to 12 minutes.

8. When done, the tops should be golden and a toothpick inserted in the middle should come out clean.
9. Allow the muffins to cool in the muffin tin for 10 minutes before removing and serving.

Nutrition:
- Calories: 267
- Protein: 4 g
- Fat: 7 g
- Carbohydrates: 8 g

Chapter 12: Easy Recipes

Berry Smoothie

Preparation Time: 5 minutes
Cooking Time: 0 minutes
Servings: 4
Ingredients:
- 1 cup berry mix (strawberries, blueberries, and cranberries)
- 4 Medjool dates, pitted and chopped
- 1-½ cups unsweetened almond milk, plus more as needed

Directions:
1. Add all the ingredients to a blender, then process until the mixture is smooth and well mixed.
2. Serve immediately or chill in the refrigerator for an hour before serving.

Nutrition:
- Calories: 473
- Fat: 4.0 g
- Carbohydrates: 103.7 g
- Fiber 9.7 g
- Protein: 14.8 g

Cranberry and Banana Smoothie

Preparation Time: 5 minutes
Cooking Time: 0 minutes
Servings: 4

Ingredients:
- 1 cup frozen cranberries
- 1 large banana, peeled
- 4 Medjool dates, pitted and chopped
- 1-½ cups unsweetened almond milk

Directions:
1. Add all the ingredients to a food processor, then process until the mixture is glossy and well mixed.
2. Serve immediately or chill in the refrigerator for an hour before serving.

Nutrition:
- Calories: 616
- Fat: 8.0 g
- Carbohydrates: 132.8 g
- Fiber 14.6 g
- Protein: 15.7 g

Spinach Cheese Flatbread Pizza

Preparation Time: 10 minutes
Cooking Time: 20 minutes
Servings: 3
Ingredients:
- 1 garlic naan flatbread
- $\frac{1}{8}$ teaspoon crushed red pepper flakes
- 2 teaspoons pesto
- 2 tablespoons feta cheese, crumbled
- 2 ounces mozzarella cheese, grated

- ¼ cup parmesan cheese, grated
- ¼ cup heavy cream
- 1 garlic clove, minced
- 1 tablespoon butter
- 5 ounces fresh spinach, chopped
- ⅛ teaspoon salt

Directions:
1. Preheat the oven to 350°Fahrenheit. Melt butter in a deep pan over medium-high heat.
2. Add spinach and garlic and saute until spinach is wilted. Add parmesan cheese, heavy cream, and salt and turn heat to low and simmer until thickened, about 5 minutes.
3. Stir frequently. Remove pan from heat and allow to cool. Spread spinach mixture on flatbread and top with feta cheese and mozzarella cheese.
4. Drizzle with pesto and bake in a preheated oven for 12 minutes. Serve.

Nutrition:
- Calories: 250
- Carbohydrates: 25 g
- Protein: 5 g
- Fat: 8 g
- Fiber 1 g

Fluffy Deep-Dish Pizza

Preparation Time: 10 minutes
Cooking Time: 2 hours
Servings: 6
Ingredients:
- 12 inch frozen whole-wheat pizza crust, thawed
- 1 medium-sized red bell pepper, cored and sliced
- 5 ounces spinach leaves, chopped
- 1 small red onion, peeled and chopped
- 1-½ teaspoons minced garlic
- ¼ teaspoon salt
- ½ teaspoon red pepper flakes
- ½ teaspoon dried thyme
- ¼ cup chopped basil, fresh
- 14 ounces pizza sauce
- 1 cup shredded vegan mozzarella

Directions:
1. Place a medium-sized non-stick skillet pan over average heat, add the oil and let it heat.
2. Add the onion, garlic and let it cook for 5 minutes or until it gets soft.
3. Then add the red bell pepper and continue cooking for 4 minutes or until it becomes tender-crisp.

4. Add the spinach, salt, red pepper, thyme, basil, and stir properly.
5. Cool off for 3 to 5 minutes or until the spinach leaves wilts, and then set it aside until it is called for.
6. Grease a 4-quarts slow cooker with a non-stick cooking spray and insert the pizza crust in it.
7. Press the dough into the bottom and spread 1 inch up along the sides.
8. Spread it with the pizza sauce, cover it with the spinach mixture and then garnish evenly with the cheese.
9. Sprinkle it with red pepper flakes, basil leaves and cover it with the lid.
10. Plugin the slow cooker and let it cook for 1-½ hours to 2 hours at the low heat setting or until the crust turns golden brown and the cheese melts completely.
11. When done, transfer the pizza to the cutting board, let it rest for 10 minutes, then slice to serve.

Nutrition:
- Calories: 250 Carbohydrates: 25 g
- Protein: 5 g
- Fat: 8 g
- Fiber 1 g

Vegetable Medley

Preparation Time: 20 minutes
Cooking Time: 15 minutes
Servings: 1
Ingredients:
- 1 tomato (diced)
- A pinch garlic pepper seasoning
- 2 fresh mushrooms (sliced)
- 2 yellow squash (cubed)
- Cooking spray
- 2 zucchini (cubed)

Directions:
1. Start by taking a large skillet and greasing it using the cooking spray. Place the skillet over medium flame and add in the tomatoes.
2. Let the tomatoes cook for about 5 minutes. Add in the garlic pepper seasoning. Toss in the mushrooms, zucchini, and squash. Let them cook on a medium flame for about 15 minutes. Serve.

Nutrition:
- Calories: 49
- Carbohydrates: 1 g
- Fat: 5 g
- Protein: 0 g

White Beans with Collard Greens

Preparation Time: 15 minutes
Cooking Time: 40 minutes
Servings: 1
Ingredients:

- 2 tablespoons water
- 1-¼ cups onion (chopped)
- 3 tablespoons garlic (minced)
- 1 cube vegetarian bouillon (beef-flavored)
- 7 ounces collard greens (chopped)
- 14-½ ounces diced tomatoes, no added salt (1 can)
- 1-¼ cups water
- Salt, to taste
- Black pepper (freshly ground), to taste
- 14-½ ounce great northern beans (1 can)
- 1 teaspoon white sugar

Directions:

1. Start by placing a large non-stick skillet on medium flame. Pour in 2 tablespoons of water. Let it heat through.
2. Stir in garlic and onion and cook for about 10 minutes. Add in more water if required to avoid scorching. Add the vegetarian bouillon to the pan. Keep stirring.
3. Toss in the collard greens and tomatoes to the onion mixture. Also, add 1-¼ cups of water.
4. Season the mixture with pepper and salt. Cover with a lid and cook for about 20 minutes. Make sure all vegetables become tender.
5. Now add in the sugar and beans and cook for about 10 minutes. Serve.

Nutrition:

- Calories: 251
- Carbohydrates: 39 g
- Fat: 3 g
- Protein: 19 g

Pumpkin Smoothie

Preparation Time: 5 minutes
Cooking Time: 0 minutes
Servings: 5
Ingredients:

- ½ cup pumpkin puree
- 4 Medjool dates, pitted and chopped
- 1 cup unsweetened almond milk
- ¼ teaspoon vanilla extract
- ¼ teaspoon ground cinnamon
- ½ cup ice
- A pinch ground nutmeg

Directions:

1. Add all the ingredients to a blender, then process until the mixture is glossy and well mixed.
2. Serve immediately.

Nutrition:

- Calories: 417
- Fat: 3.0 g
- Carbohydrates: 94.9 g
- Fiber 10.4 g
- Protein: 11.4 g

Super Smoothie

Preparation Time: 5 minutes
Cooking Time: 0 minutes
Servings: 4
Ingredients:

- 1 banana, peeled
- 1 cup chopped mango
- 1 cup raspberries
- ¼ cup rolled oats
- 1 carrot, peeled
- 1 cup chopped fresh kale
- 2 tablespoons chopped fresh parsley
- 1 tablespoon flaxseeds
- 1 tablespoon grated fresh ginger
- ½ cup unsweetened soy milk
- 1 cup water

Directions:

1. Put all the ingredients in a food processor, then blitz until glossy and smooth.
2. Serve immediately or chill in the refrigerator for an hour before serving.

Nutrition:

- Calories: 550
- Fat: 39.0 g
- Carbohydrates: 31.0 g
- Fiber 15.0 g
- Protein: 13.0 g

Cookie Dough

Preparation Time: 25 minutes
Cooking Time: 0 minutes
Servings: 18-20
Ingredients:

- 8 tablespoons unsalted grass-fed butter, at room temperature
- ⅓ cup swerve sweetener
- ½ teaspoon vanilla extract
- ¼ teaspoon salt
- 2 cups almond flour
- ½ cup dark chocolate chips

Directions:

1. In the bowl of a stand mixer, combine the butter, swerve, vanilla, and salt. Beat until the mixture is light and fluffy.
2. Add the almond flour and continue to mix on low until a dough forms. Fold in the chocolate chips until just barely combined.
3. Place the dough in the refrigerator for about 15 minutes to set. Line a baking sheet with parchment paper.
4. Using a 2-inch cookie scoop, scoop balls of dough onto the prepared baking sheet. Store the cookie dough balls in the refrigerator until ready to eat.

Nutrition:

- Calories: 122
- Fat: 10 g
- Protein: 2 g
- Carbohydrates: 6 g

No-Bake Coconut Cookies

Preparation Time: 40 minutes
Cooking Time: 5 minutes
Servings: 12
Ingredients:

- 2 tablespoons grass-fed butter
- $^2/_3$ cup crunchy natural peanut butter
- 1-½ tablespoons unsweetened cocoa powder
- 5 or 6 drops liquid stevia
- 1 cup finely shredded unsweetened coconut flakes

Directions:

1. Line a baking sheet with parchment paper. Dissolve the butter in a medium saucepan over medium heat. Add the peanut butter and cocoa powder, and stir well.
2. Remove from the heat and add the stevia. Stir in the coconut flakes and mix until all the ingredients are well combined.
3. Scoop the dough in a small spoonful onto the prepared baking sheet. Put the baking sheet in the refrigerator within 30 minutes to set. Serve.

Nutrition:

- Calories: 153
- Fat: 13 g
- Protein: 4 g
- Carbohydrates: 5 g

Lemon Bars

Preparation Time: 15 minutes
Cooking Time: 25 minutes
Servings: 9
Ingredients:

- 1-$^1/_8$ cups almond flour
- $^1/_8$ cup powdered erythritol sweetener, plus $^2/_3$ cup, plus more for sprinkling
- $^1/_3$ cup coconut oil, melted
- 2 large organic eggs
- 2 tablespoons freshly squeezed lemon juice
- ¼ teaspoon baking powder
- ½ tablespoon coconut flour

Directions:

1. Preheat the oven to 350°Fahrenheit. Oil an 8-by-8-inch baking dish with cooking spray. In a small bowl, combine the almond flour and $^1/_8$ cup of erythritol. Add the melted coconut oil and blend until the mixture is crumbly.
2. Put the crust batter to press into the bottom of the prepared baking dish. Bake within 10 minutes, or until the crust is slightly golden brown.
3. In a high-powered blender, combine the eggs, remaining $^2/_3$ cup of erythritol, lemon juice, baking powder, and coconut flour. Then blend for about 30 seconds.
4. Put the filling into the crust and cook for an additional 10 to 12 minutes, or until the filling is set. Remove from the oven and sprinkle with a dusting of powdered sweetener. Allow to cool, then serve.

Nutrition:

- Calories: 128
- Fat: 12 g
- Protein: 3 g
- Carbohydrates: 2 g

Peanut Butter Cookies

Preparation Time: 10 minutes
Cooking Time: 10 minutes
Servings: 12
Ingredients:

- 1 cup chunky natural peanut butter
- ¾ cup erythritol, granulated
- 1 organic egg, beaten

Directions:

1. Preheat the oven to 350°Fahrenheit. Oil a baking sheet with cooking spray. Combine the peanut butter and erythritol in a medium mixing bowl. Mix well.
2. Add the egg and stir until thoroughly combined. Using a 2-inch cookie scoop, roll the dough into balls and set them on the prepared baking sheet.
3. Using the back of a fork, press a crisscross pattern onto the top of each cookie. Bake for 9

to 10 minutes, then transfer to a wire rack to cool.

Nutrition:
- Calories: 135
- Fat: 11 g
- Protein: 5 g
- Carbohydrates: 4 g

Fudge Brownies

Preparation Time: 15 minutes
Cooking Time: 20 minutes
Servings: 12
Ingredients:
- 12 tablespoons (1-½ sticks) grass-fed butter
- 2 ounces dark chocolate squares (80 percent or higher), broken into chunks
- ¼ cup unsweetened cocoa powder
- ½ cup almond flour
- $^2/_3$ cup swerve sweetener
- ½ teaspoon baking powder
- 3 large organic eggs, beaten

Directions:
1. Warm your oven to 350°Fahrenheit. Oil an 8-by-8-inch baking dish with cooking spray. In a small saucepan over low heat, melt the butter and dark chocolate while stirring.
2. When melted, add the cocoa powder and stir until combined. Set aside. In a small mixing bowl, combine the almond flour, swerve, and baking powder. Stir well.
3. In a separate bowl, pour in the eggs and then slowly stir in the dark chocolate mixture. Mix together for about 1 minute to make sure everything is well combined.
4. Pour the flour mixture into the chocolate mixture and stir until a batter forms. Spread the batter into the prepared baking dish and cook for 18 to 20 minutes, or until a toothpick inserted into the center comes out clean.
5. Remove then allow to cool before cutting into 12 squares.

Nutrition:
- Calories: 163 Fat: 15 g
- Protein: 3 g Carbohydrates: 4 g

Vegan Eggplant Patties

Preparation Time: 30 minutes
Cooking Time: 15 minutes
Servings: 6
Ingredients:
- 2 big eggplants
- 1 onion finely diced
- 1 tablespoon smashed garlic cloves
- 1 bunch raw parsley, chopped
- ½ cup almond meal
- 4 tablespoons Kalamata olives, pitted and sliced
- 1 tablespoon baking soda
- Salt and ground pepper to taste
- Olive oil or avocado oil, for frying

Directions:
1. Peel off eggplants, rinse, and cut in half. Saute eggplant cubes in a non-stick skillet, occasionally stirring, for about 10 minutes.
2. Transfer to a large bowl and mash with an immersion blender. Add eggplant puree into a bowl and add in all remaining ingredients (except oil).
3. Knead a mixture using your hands until the dough is smooth, sticky, and easy to shape. Shape mixture into 6 patties.
4. Heat up the olive oil in a frying skillet on medium-high heat. Fry patties for about 3 to 4 minutes per side. Remove patties on a platter lined with kitchen paper towel to drain. Serve warm.

Nutrition:
- Calories: 210
- Carbohydrates: 16 g
- Fat: 12 g
- Protein: 8 g

Spinach Chips

Preparation Time: 10 minutes
Cooking Time: 20 minutes
Servings: 4
Ingredients:
- 1 pound baby spinach, well dried
- Salt and black pepper to taste
- ½ teaspoon oregano, dried
- 1 teaspoon sweet paprika
- Cooking spray

Directions:
1. Oiled a baking sheet using cooking spray and spread the spinach leaves on it. Add the other ingredients, toss gently, and bake at 435°Fahrenheit for 20 minutes.
2. Serve as a snack.

Nutrition:
- Calories: 140 Fat: 4.2 g
- Carbohydrates: 6 g Protein: 4 g

Balsamic Zucchini Bowls

Preparation Time: 10 minutes
Cooking Time: 3 hours
Servings: 8
Ingredients:
- 3 zucchinis, thinly sliced
- Salt and black pepper to taste
- 2 tablespoons olive oil
- 1 teaspoon turmeric powder
- 1 teaspoon coriander, ground
- 2 tablespoons balsamic vinegar

Directions:
1. Spread the zucchini on a lined baking sheet and mix it with the other ingredients.
2. Toss and bake at 360°Fahrenheit for 3 hours.
3. Divide into bowls and serve as a snack.

Nutrition:
- Calories: 100
- Fat: 3 g
- Carbohydrates: 3 g
- Protein: 4.5 g

Protein: Raffaello Candies

Preparation Time: 15 minutes
Cooking Time: 0 minutes
Servings: 12
Ingredients:
- 1-½ cups desiccated coconut flakes
- ½ cup coconut butter softened
- 4 tablespoons coconut milk canned
- 4 teaspoons coconut palm sugar (or granulated sugar)
- 1 teaspoon pure vanilla extract
- 1 tablespoon vegan protein powder (pea or soy)
- 15 whole almonds

Directions:
1. Put 1 cup of desiccated coconut flakes, and all remaining ingredients in the blender (except almonds), and blend until soft. If your dough is too thick, add some coconut milk.
2. In a bowl, add remaining coconut flakes. Coat every almond in one tablespoon of mixture and roll into a ball. Roll each ball in coconut flakes. Chill in the fridge for several hours.

Nutrition:
- Calories: 155
- Carbohydrates: 9 g
- Fat: 12 g
- Protein: 2 g

Protein:-Rich Pumpkin Bowl

Preparation Time: 10 minutes
Cooking Time: 0 minutes
Servings: 2
Ingredients:
- 1-½ cups almond milk
- 1 cup pumpkin puree canned, with salt
- ½ cup chopped walnuts
- 1 scoop vegan soy protein powder
- 1 teaspoon pure vanilla extract
- A handful cacao nibs

Directions:
1. Add all ingredients in a blender apart from the cacao nibs. Blend until smooth. Serve in bowls and sprinkle with cacao nibs.

Nutrition:
- Calories: 140
- Carbohydrates: 17 g
- Fat: 7 g
- Protein: 1 g

Red Potato-Garlic Balls

Preparation Time: 40 minutes
Cooking Time: 25 minutes
Servings: 4
Ingredients:
- 1-½ pounds red potatoes
- 3 garlic cloves finely chopped
- 1 tablespoon fresh finely chopped parsley
- ¼ teaspoon ground turmeric
- Salt and ground pepper to taste

Directions:
1. Rinse potatoes and place unpeeled into a large pot. Pour water to cover potatoes and bring to boil. Cook for about 20 to 25 minutes on medium heat.
2. Rinse potatoes and let them cool down. Peel potatoes and mash them; add finely chopped garlic, and salt and pepper.
3. Form the potato mixture into small balls. Sprinkle with chopped parsley and refrigerate for several hours.
4. Serve.

Nutrition:
- Calories: 212 Carbohydrates: 30 g
- Fat: 8 g Protein: 3 g

Steamed Broccoli with Sesame

Preparation Time: 15 minutes
Cooking Time: 5 minutes
Servings: 2

Ingredients:

- 1-½ pounds fresh broccoli florets
- ½ cup sesame oil
- 4 tablespoons sesame seeds
- Salt and ground pepper to taste

Directions:

1. Put broccoli florets in your steamer basket above boiling water. Cover and steam for about 4 to 5 minutes. Remove from steam and place broccoli in serving the dish.
2. Season with salt and pepper, and drizzle with sesame oil; toss to coat. Sprinkle with sesame seeds and serve immediately.

Nutrition:

- Calories: 54
- Carbohydrates: 5 g
- Fat: 2 g
- Protein: 3 g

Mediterranean Marinated Olives

Preparation Time: 10 minutes
Cooking Time: 0 minutes

Servings: 2
Ingredients:

- 24 large olives, black, green, Kalamata
- ½ cup extra-virgin olive oil
- 4 garlic cloves, thinly sliced
- 2 tablespoons fresh lemon juice
- 2 teaspoons coriander seeds, crushed
- ½ teaspoon crushed red pepper
- 1 teaspoon dried thyme
- 1 teaspoon dried rosemary, crushed
- Salt and ground pepper to taste

Directions:

1. Place olives and all remaining fixings in a large container or bag, and shake to combine well.
2. Cover and refrigerate to marinate overnight.
3. Serve.

Nutrition:

- Calories: 47
- Carbohydrates: 1 g
- Fat: 4 g
- Protein: 0 g

Conclusion

Now that you've read through all these recipes and reviews of excellent vegan meals and snacks, you should be armed with enough tips to last you a lifetime. You need never worry about not having something to eat again because there are so many options for both vegans and those who are just making the gradual transition.

If you have any major health concerns about whether or not a plant-based diet is good for you, talk to your doctor or a nutritionist.

Also, be aware that certain diets are not suitable for certain religions. If you're a Buddhist or Muslim, the animal rights issues might create some conflict in your meal choices. For example, if you're not allowed to eat pork, then bacon will be out of the question. If anything prevents you from eating something vital to your dietary needs, try to find an alternative.

At the very least, remove one animal at a time from your diet until you're finally eating strictly plant-based foods. That way you'll find out which animal created the most dilemma for you and where it's easier to make those changes.

If you're a vegan, please feel free to share your recipes in our comments section and enjoy everyone else's recipes! Please let us know if there are other things that we didn't cover or if you find some shocking information or something unusual (like eggplant ice cream). The more knowledge we can share, the better off we all are!

So, now comes the moment of truth (to mix my metaphors). What are you going to make with your newfound knowledge? After all, your body is a temple, and what better way to honor it than by filling it with healthy food that nourishes you from the inside out.

Just think about how much healthier you can be if you fill your body with the right things. You can live longer and have more energy to do the things you love. Maybe even cheat death completely. What a thought!

So why not give it a try for at least 30 days? Like most people, you'll find that eating vegan is really easy and fun too! In fact, once you get started, it will become second nature before long.

Especially if you're on the fence like me, the dozens of reviews and recipes from others that you'll find here should undoubtedly make it much easier for you to make the transition. Even with all those options, even my family members have been impressed with how delicious the vegan dishes are!

So go ahead and re-enjoy your cuisine while giving your body a break.

That is something that each of us is entitled to.

Made in the USA
Monee, IL
19 December 2022

23008839R00063